Rosie Dimand.

Postnatal Depression

A Guide for Health Professionals

John L. Cox

MA DM FRCP (Ed) DPM MRCPsych

Professor of Psychiatry, Department of Postgraduate
Medicine, University of Keele, Staffordshire;
formerly Senior Lecturer, Department of Psychiatry,
University of Edinburgh; Honorary Consultant,
Royal Edinburgh Hospital and Western General
Hospital, Edinburgh

Foreword by

Brice Pitt
MD FRCPsych

Consultant Psychiatrist, The London Hospital

Churchill Livingstone ▦

EDINBURGH LONDON MELBOURNE AND NEW YORK 1986

CHURCHILL LIVINGSTONE
Medical Division of Longman Group Limited

Distributed in the United States of America by
Churchill Livingstone Inc., 1560 Broadway, New York,
N. Y. 10036, and by associated companies, branches
and representatives throughout the world.

First published 1986

ISBN 0 443 03178 9

British Library Cataloguing in Publication Data
Cox, John L.
    Postnatal depression: a guide for health
    professionals.
    1. Postpartum depression
    I. Title
    618.7   RG852

Library of Congress Cataloging in Publication Data
Cox, John L. (John Lee)
    Postnatal depression.
    Includes index.
    1. Postpartum psychiatric disorders. 2. Postpartum
psychiatric disorders — Social aspects. 3. Postpartum
psychiatric disorders — Research. I. Title. [DNLM:
1. Depression. 2. Depressive Disorder. 3. Psychotic Disorders.
4. Puerperal Disorders. WQ 500 C877p]
RG850.C69   1986   616.85'27   85–22331

Produced by Longman Singapore Publishers (Pte) Ltd.
Printed in Singapore.

Foreword

Major mental disorder arising shortly after childbirth has intrigued psychiatrists (and their predecessors) for many years — indeed as far back as the days of Hippocrates. Debates about whether 'postpartum psychosis' is a specific entity have been stimulating, and while it is now widely accepted that these are the same sorts of mental disorders as develop at other times, there are enough special features to excite continuing speculation.

Still more interesting, though, is the clear evidence that child-birth is a mighty precipitating factor in those who are genetically and constitutionally predisposed to major mental illness. We are very much clearer about what happens than why, and our powers of prevention are as yet puny. Well before the spate of bonding literature, a policy of admitting babies with their mentally sick mothers was well established in Britain, and assumed to be a 'good thing', but this policy has never, to my knowledge, been evaluated by comparison with one where mother and baby are separated.

Less severe puerperal mental disorders were largely ignored until about 20 years ago, and though there are many studies demonstrating their high prevalence and distressing effects in the short-and the long-term, it appears, from Dr Cox's recent investigations, that for practical purposes they are still largely ignored. As one of the earlier workers in this recently opened field I find it dispiriting and perplexing that such a common and troublesome problem as postnatal depression is not yet widely recognised or treated properly. One would have thought that by now it would at least be a feminist issue. As it is, far too many women — and their families — appear to suffer in relative silence.

Nevertheless, research has grown apace, and though most has been British, the timely formation of a special interest group — the Marcé Society (named after the French psychiatrist whose pioneering 19th century studies of women with mental illness related to pregnancy and childbirth were made known to modern readers by the first President, Jim Hamilton) — has helped international investigation and understanding.

There is still much that we need to know. Although risk factors for postnatal depression have been identified, the profile of vulnerability is far less well-defined than for puerperal psychosis: all we know for sure is that at least 1 in 10 new mothers will get it. We know that most sufferers do not get treated, but not what treatments are effective. We know a good deal less about the effects of the disorder a year or more later than we do of its early symptoms. We also very much want to know about cultural factors, and here Dr Cox's unique experience in Uganda offers an unusual and instructive perspective.

I recall with pleasure a happy time when Dr Cox, Dr Stephen Wolkind and I were all working in the Department of Psychiatry at the London Hospital, in very different areas — general psychiatry, child psychiatry and psychogeriatrics — but sharing a fascination with the psychiatry of childbirth.

The germ of a book was sown at that time. We went our separate ways, but all went on, though individually, to write a book about this pet topic.

Dr Cox's is the last to appear, and very welcome. Since his return from Africa he has moved to Edinburgh which is now a particularly fruitful source of research, not least into postnatal problems, and this is reflected in the book. For me it is most valuable for its account of the evolution of such research and its clear description of methods. The Edinburgh Postnatal Depression Scale may prove a valuable screening instrument in further studies.

However, this is by no means a purely academic, though it is a scholarly, work. There is manifest concern for mothers who suffer needlessly and an almost evangelical zeal to improve matters to which I warm.

I hope, therefore, that the book will be read not only by the wide range of professionals concerned with childbirth, but also by the consumers of their services and their families.

Brice Pitt

Acknowledgements

This book is a distillation of collaborative clinical and research work that has extended for almost 15 years and I am therefore greatly indebted to my professional colleagues, as well as to the childbearing women who so willingly described their life histories to us. In particular the Ugandan study would not have been possible without the initial encouragement of Sir Desmond Pond, Professor Allen German and Dr John Orley, as well as the practical assistance from Sister Lwanga, Eunice Sendagira, Charles Kimbugwe and Mrs Karin Cox at Kasangati Health Centre. My special thanks also to Professor R. E. Kendell, Mr R. J. McGuire, Dr R. Kumar, Miss Y. Connor, Ms J. Holden, Ms A. Rooney, Dr R. Wrate, Dr R. Sagovsky, Dr P. Thomas, Ms I. Henderson and Dr P. Holland for their research collaboration and for their many interesting discussions. I am also grateful to Dr Brice Pitt, Dr C. Platz, and Professor Kendell for their helpful comments on the manuscript, and for Dr Pitt's ready agreement to write the Foreword. His pioneer work has indeed stimulated others to investigate further the puerperal mood disorders. Finally my most sincere thanks to my secretary, Mrs Marjory Dodd, for her unremitting professional assistance, her forbearance with my adjusted drafts and her overall encouragement with a task that otherwise might not have been completed, or even initiated.

John Cox

To Karin and our daughters, Christina, Ann-Marie and Susanne, without whose help this book would not have been written.

Contents

1

Introduction

In the last decade the diagnosis of postnatal depression has become of increased concern to community health professionals as well as to hospital specialists, and the general public is also now more aware that such depression can cause much personal and family distress.

Hitherto doctors, health visitors and midwives could recall an occasional mother who developed a puerperal psychosis that was treated by a psychiatrist but were less familiar with the puerperal depression that occurred in the community.

It is one aim of this book therefore to make more available to community health professionals, as well as to hospital specialists, recent research findings about the frequency, causation and management of postnatal depression. It is now known for example that one in seven women who attend a postnatal or baby clinic may be suffering from such a depressive illness and that careful assessment of such mothers is therefore most important (Cox et al, 1982). Our clinical and research experience has also shown that many such depressed mothers were not always identified by primary care workers as having an illness that required specific treatment. Because of the close medical scrutiny of mothers following childbirth, which may include entry to a home even when a mother has not requested such a visit, it is a sad paradox that many depressed mothers are not identified.

The reasons for this seeming neglect of psychiatric complications in the puerperium are complex and include the lack of educational textbooks, as well as the inaccessibility of the psychiatric literature. Thus, whilst Margaret Myles' (1985) *Textbook for Midwives* now includes a brief section on puerperal mood disorders, this topic is not comprehensively covered in other obstetric textbooks, and one recent book for obstetricians failed to mention puerperal depression at all.

It is my hope, therefore, that this book will contribute to postnatal care by making information about postnatal depression more available to doctors and other health workers, and that these health professionals will then be encouraged to make this important diagnosis. Most research findings also underline the scientific credibility of the concern shown by women themselves; the collaboration between self-help groups and health workers has already assisted substantially to disseminate knowledge about puerperal mental illness and also to motivate scientific researchers.

The increased awareness of the general public about postnatal depression is also apparent and has followed the publication of books by Pitt (1978), Welburn (1980) and Dalton (1980), as well as radio programmes and documentary films on television. It is now indeed more widely recognised that childbirth is not always followed by months of happiness or contentment. This media coverage has also challenged another belief that postnatal depression is only a trivial disorder that can be readily dismissed as 'just the blues'.

The front cover of Vivienne Welburn's book, *Postnatal Depression*, for example, which shows a young depressed mother with downcast eyes closely holding her small baby, strikes a cord for many women who readily personalize the poignant dilemma illustrated by the quotation:

> you have to go around with that big smile on your face, with people saying 'aren't you lucky to have such a dear little baby' and you feel utter despair.

Indeed it is this culturally-sanctioned belief that a mother should be happy after childbirth that may exacerbate further her already low self-esteem, and so perpetuate or even initiate a more serious depressive illness.

This book attempts to bridge this large educational gap between what is now known about postnatal depression, and what is commonly taught to students, and so to make more available to primary care workers and hospital specialists research findings, as well as clinical observations of this common puerperal mood disorder. It is hoped that this information will counteract the belief that the present interest in postnatal depression is 'a fuss about nothing', and will also show that the women's own concern about the plight of such depressed mothers is a fully legitimate 'cry for help'.

Sociocultural aspects of postnatal depression are given particular importance in Chapter 3, because a full understanding of this disorder is only grasped if the local social and cultural matrix of the mother and her family are understood. Puerperal depression follows the childbirth 'event' which has wide implications for the whole society, and not just for the local family.

In other chapters I have brought together research findings from studies carried out in the UK and Africa which have increased knowledge about the frequency and presentation of postnatal depression, and provided scientific facts of particular importance if a full appreciation of this subject is to be gained.

In some countries the subject of postnatal depression has become so controversial that mothers demand the right to be treated with progesterone by their doctor, and in the UK many women clearly articulate the belief that one cause of postnatal depression is the change in role for women in present day society. However other possible causal factors of postnatal depression include the contribution of disturbed family relationships, the vulnerability of the mother's personality as well as that of her husband, and biological variables such as hormonal changes. Chapter 5 describes how postnatal depression may present to a health visitor or a general practitioner, and how it is diagnosed and treated.

The major depressive psychoses are briefly outlined in Chapter 6, which also discusses the need for a mother and baby unit, the role of the social worker, as well as the contribution of community psychiatric nurses and health visitors in the management of these more severely disturbed mothers. The recognition and management of postnatal blues are included in Chapter 7; the prevention of postnatal depression is described in Chapter 8.

This guide then concludes by bringing together these diverse aspects of postnatal depression, and emphasises the need for greater and more prolonged multiprofessional collaboration if this disorder is to be identified more effectively, and its causation to be more adequately understood.

REFERENCES

Cox J L, Connor Y M, Kendell R E 1982 Prospective study of the psychiatric
    disorders of childbirth. British Journal of Psychiatry 140: 111-117
Dalton K 1980 Depression after childbirth. Oxford University Press, Oxford
Myles M 1985 Textbook for midwives, 10th edn. Churchill Livingstone, Edinburgh
Pitt B 1978 Feelings about childbirth. Sheldon Press, London
Welburn V 1980 Postnatal depression. Fontana Books, London

2

Sociocultural aspects of postnatal depression

INTRODUCTION

It is not surprising that most societies throughout the world, irrespective of their language and customs, attach particular importance to illnesses and misfortunes associated with childbirth, because this is a 'life event' that not only creates a new generation but is also of immediate importance to the mother and her family. Thus Mead & Newton (1967), in their comprehensive survey of childbirth customs, found that many cultures patterned the behaviour of individuals and groups associated with the process of reproduction and that pregnancy was rarely ignored altogether.

Indeed over 2000 years ago Hippocrates specifically described women with puerperal mental illness, and postulated that physiological factors such as milk diverted from the breast to the brain, or the suppression of locheal discharge were important causes.

These physiological explanations for puerperal mental illness were not generally fashionable in the Middle Ages when a depressed mother was more likely to be regarded as a witch, or her illness believed to be caused by witchcraft. A vivid account of such 'projective systems' has been given by Cohn (1975) who describes how witches were believed to eat small babies, as well as attend witches' Sabbaths.

It is also of interest to consider the categories of puerperal mental illness that were used in an African society before Western doctors arrived with Western classifications of psychiatric disturbance. Thus the Ganda, the largest tribe in Uganda, have a traditional puerperal mental illness called 'Amakiro', which has been recognised for at least a century. The cause of Amakiro is somewhat different from the usual explanation given for a Western puerperal psychosis; the illness is thought to be caused by a mother's promiscuity during pregnancy. In contemporary times Amakiro is still regarded as a non-Western illness and a mother with Amakiro is usually taken for treatment to a traditional healer and would not initially seek help from a Western trained doctor. The symptom most commonly reported of Amakiro is that a mother wants to eat her baby, but other symptoms more familiar to a Western observer, include restlessness, mental confusion and pallor (Orley, 1970; Cox, 1979).

In Nigeria there is also a traditional postnatal mental illness 'Abisiwin' which, unlike Amakiro, is thought to be caused not by undesirable behaviour of the mother during pregnancy, but by excessive bodily heat; a common explanation for other disorders in Nigeria.

It seems likely that these African societies, as in a Western society, have recognised certain distinctive features or social consequences of mental illness that follow childbirth, and have therefore given a specific name to these disorders. Interestingly, ideas of a mother wishing to incorporate her baby are familiar to psychoanalysts such as Winnicott (1949), who recognise in a mother's primary cannibalistic impulse frustration that she cannot eat her baby nor 'trade in sex' with him.

It might be expected that these popular beliefs about the cause of puerperal mental illness will reflect the current preoccupations of a society. Thus at a time when psychoanalysis was a popular psychological theory, puerperal psychoses were commonly thought to be caused by a suppression of sexuality, or to protect against latent homosexual desires. In more recent years, when psychoanalytic theory is less influential, there is greater interest in possible biological explanations, such as changes in hormone levels. The cause of postnatal depression is also linked to concern about excessive medicalisation of childbearing, whether childbirth should be in hospital or at home, the changing roles of women and the loss of family support due to increased mobility. It can therefore be difficult to discuss the aetiology of postnatal depression without being influenced by such legitimate social preoccupations.

McIntyre (1977) has provided a succinct critique of popular views of the aetiology of postnatal depression, and criticised Arms (1975) and Shaw (1974) who compared the apparent disadvantages of modern childbirth practice, thought to predispose to postnatal depression, with what childbirth was like previously in a Western society, or as it is presently thought to be in a 'primitive' society. These authors put forward the opinion that, before the development of modern obstetric practice, childbirth was not associated with pain or suffering. A similar attitude was also discussed in a review of cultural aspects of postnatal depression by Stern & Crookman (1983), when the hypothesis was advocated that postnatal depression was a culture-bound Western syndrome which was unlikely to occur in a non-Western society.

The limitations of these generalisations is illustrated by a consideration of postpartum taboos, and the evidence that postnatal depression is indeed readily identifiable in a traditional African society.

POSTPARTUM TABOOS

Many societies have definite rules governing how a mother should behave in the 40 days that follow childbirth. In Jamaica, for example, a period of ritual seclusion follows childbirth which is particularly intense for the first nine nights, and Kitzinger (1982) describes this as similar to the seclusion that follows a bereavement. This is followed by a secondary, but less restricted, seclusion for a further 31 nights, when the mother remains at home with her baby and is looked after by her own mother. In India, among the lower Hindu castes, a postpartum woman is regarded as impure for 40 days and during this time she and her child should not come out of confinement. In a gypsy community, Oakley (1975) reports that childbirth is polluting, and to prevent contamination cooking is carried out by other women, or by older children. Among Punjabi women living in Britain the length of the confinement after childbirth varies, and depends on whether other women in the household can help, as well as on economic considerations (Homans, 1982). In China the postpartum period is referred to as 'doing the month', when extra attention is given to the mother by her family, as well as by her wider social network.

Postnatal rituals, however, are also found in contemporary Western countries. There is, for example, a similar 6-week period after childbirth when special observation of the mother is carried out that is enshrined in present day obstetric practice. The post-natal clinic usually takes place after 6 weeks and is customarily regarded as a signal that full domestic and marital responsibilities should be resumed. It is also of interest that a baptism, which may be regarded as a public statement about the place of the child within the family as well as a Christian ceremony, also takes place at about this time.

It is not my intention however to review further the socio-anthropological literature of postpartum taboos, a task already carried out by others (see Mead & Newton, 1972; Stern & Crookman, 1983; MacCormack, 1982). My more limited intention is to point out that the diagnostic labels used to describe postnatal mental illness, as well as the timing of postpartum clinical interventions and the extra attention given to childbearing mothers, are all linked to the sociocultural attitudes towards the parturant mother who is regarded as being especially vulnerable.

different attitudes towards postpartum mothers.

CHILDBEARING AND TRADITIONAL BELIEFS IN UGANDA

In planning the African study of postnatal depression, I was assisted considerably by Roscoe (1908) who had described the customs of Ganda society related to childbearing, and observed the importance attached to reproduction. Every married woman, he said, was 'anxious to become a mother' and was 'expected' to show signs of maternity within a few weeks of marriage; a child-less woman was despised and became a 'slave and drudge of the household'.

Other examples of the intense feeling of the family for the satisfactory growth of the child are described; the husband may ask a relative to live in his house to look after his wife while she is pregnant and must also ensure that certain taboos, such as not allowing a man to step over her legs, are observed. The woman herself must not step over a mat or over the feet of another man; if she sat in a doorway when a man entered it was believed that the fetus would die. Another example of society's concern for the well-being of the child is the belief that a pregnant woman should not look at an unhealthy child, or laugh at a lame man, because a misfortune might happen.

Childbirth in Ganda society usually took place outside the house in the banana grove and was assisted by relatives, and often by a traditional midwife. A prolonged or difficult labour was particularly stressful for the mother because any such difficulty was believed to be brought about by her own immorality, and a mother who experienced such difficulties during labour was urged to confess her previous misdeeds.

Thus in Ganda society the legitimacy of the baby was of particular importance, and only when this legitimacy was fully established could the child be named, and so placed in a family or clan; the ceremony to determine the legitimacy of the child was of much importance. Legitimacy was even determined before birth during a ceremony in which the mother was examined by members of her husband's clan and then inspected for a second time the following morning when her husband jumped over her. It was believed that if this ceremony was carried out satisfactorily, an illegitimate fetus would die.

After birth a yet more complicated ceremony took place to re-establish legitimacy; the mother first passed the umbilical cord to her mother-in-law who placed it in a large vessel which contained beer, milk and water. If the umbilical cord floated, the baby was declared to be fully legitimate. The midwife, who was of crucial importance to the success of this ceremony, could, by rubbing the umbilical cord with fat, assist it to float and so confirm the baby's legitimacy.

Sterility carried much social stigma, and barrenness was thought to be caused by a traditional disease called Ekigolanga. Bennett (1965) described the symptoms of this illness, which included abdominal pain and a thin voice. Barrenness was thought to be brought about by a bad spirit from another person.

It is clear that an understanding of these traditional beliefs may help us to understand certain aspects of puerperal mood disorder, and also illustrate the need of societies to give special attention to the childbearing women, and particularly to illnesses and misfortunes that occur after childbirth.

Sociocultural differences

During the planning stage of my study of postnatal depression in Uganda, it became clear that the sociocultural differences between African and European societies would have a major impact on the way in which the research was planned, and on the implication of any research findings. It would not have been appropriate for example to ask an African mother whether her baby was 'wanted', since childbearing was so widely regarded as desirable. Likewise a question about family planning yielded little information; contraception was not routinely used, and children were still regarded as an insurance against future misfortune. The family structure amongst the Africans was strikingly different, both with regard to the role obligations within the marriage, and the details of the marriage contract. Thus one-half of the African women had co-wives who shared in the responsibility for bringing up children; an arrangement which had certain advantages, especially if one of the wives was infertile. Most mothers lived close to their own extended family, and also gave considerable respect to their parents, and to their father in particular.

Most mothers spent a large proportion of their time looking after their own as well as others' children. They also cultivated the 'shamba' (garden) to produce bananas and sweet potatoes for their family, prepared food and carried water. Only a few mothers had a cash income. It was inappropriate to ask an African woman how she got on with her own mother or what sort of person her own mother was; such questions had no clear answers and indeed it was often apparent to the interviewer that these were regarded as strange questions because the mother did not know which relative the interviewer was referring to. The woman was uncertain whether the interviewer was referring to her biological mother, her aunt, or even to another of her father's 'co-wives.'

Despite these cultural differences, however, it *was* possible to carry out a psychiatric interview before and after childbirth to determine the present mental state, as well as establish specific sociocultural data about the family, the work and coping ability. Further details of the research method, and the results, are included in the Appendix (pp 87–93).

Our results showed that postnatal depression could be identified in an African woman, and that many symptoms were similar to those described in Europeans; feelings of self-blame and difficulty coping, however, were less commonly described. 18 (10%) of the 180 Africans had a postnatal depressive illness that usually commenced within 2 weeks of delivery. The depressive symptoms were disabling, distressing and usually lasted for several months. Six of the 18 depressed mothers were so impaired by their illness that they were unable to dig or carry water. Because one-third of the women had delivered their baby at home, rather than in the local maternity unit, we could investigate whether a home delivery was followed by less depression than a hospital delivery, but no such difference was found. Childbirth in hospital was not more likely to be followed by depression than a home delivery.

It is apparent therefore that postnatal depression does occur in an African society and is not a 'culture-bound' illness, narrowly restricted to a particular Western society. Nevertheless its symptoms are only fully understood when the specific cultural context of the mother is carefully considered.

REFERENCES

Arms S 1975 Immaculate deception: a new look at women and childbirth in America. San Francisco Book Co., Haughton, Boston

Bennett F J 1965 The social, cultural and emotional aspects of sterility in women in Buganda. Fertility and Sterility 16: 243-251

Cohn M 1975 Europe's inner demons. Chatto-Heinemann for Sussex University Press

Cox J L 1979 Amakiro: A Ugandan puerperal psychosis? Social Psychiatry 14: 49-52

Homans H 1982 Pregnancy and birth as rites of passage In: MacCormack C P (ed) Ethnography of fertility and birth. Academic Press, London

Kitzinger S 1982 The social context of birth: some comparisons between childbirth in Jamaica and Britain. In: MacCormack CP (ed) Ethnography of fertility and birth. Academic Press, London

MacCormack CP (ed) 1982 Ethnography of fertility and birth. Academic Press, London

McIntyre S 1977 Childbirth: the myth of the golden age. World Medicine June: 17-22

Mead M, Newton N 1967 Cultural patterning of perinatal behaviour in childbearing—social and psychological aspects. In: Richardson S A, Guttmacher A F, (eds) Williams and Wilkins, Baltimore

Oakley A 1975 Women confined: towards a sociology of childbirth. Martin Robertson, London

Orley J 1970 Culture and Mental illness; A Study from Uganda. Makerere institute of Social Research: East African Publishing House.

Roscoe J 1911 The Baganda. Macmillan, London

Shaw NS 1974 Forced labour; maternity care in the United States. Pergamon Press, London

Stern G, Kruckman L 1983 Multi-disciplinary on postpartum depression: an anthropological critique. Social Science and Medicine 17: 1027-1041
Winnicott D W 1949 Collected papers. Tavistock Publications, London, p 194-203

3

Research: problems and progress

PROBLEMS OF DEFINITIONS

One of the problems for the reader of articles about postnatal depression is that the word 'depression' is used in several different ways: one writer for example refers to depression as a mood state, whilst another uses the word to describe the cluster of symptoms which are sufficiently characteristic to make the diagnosis of a depressive illness. A more common difficulty, which is even more misleading, is caused by the writer who refers to 'postnatal depression' occurring in the first 2 weeks postpartum, as the reader is then uncertain whether the author is referring to postnatal blues, or the early onset of a prolonged depressive illness.

The definitions of puerperal mood disorder given below are those which are commonly used by psychiatrists as well as by other mental health specialists.

Postnatal depression

This psychiatric diagnosis should be restricted to mothers with a depressive illness who do not usually have false beliefs (delusions), or experience sensations in the absence of a stimulus (hallucinations), and who do not usually need immediate treatment in a psychiatric hospital. In postnatal depression, behaviour is not therefore obviously abnormal, and a mother may appear to have no personal difficulties at all. Only careful enquiry about the presence or absence of certain depressive symptoms will enable this disorder to be recognised.

Postnatal depression as defined above is similar to the first descriptions by Pitt (1968) of mothers with unfamiliar and prolonged depressive symptoms, which usually commenced after the mother returned home, lasted for several weeks and also caused distress to herself as well as to her family. The symptoms of postnatal depression, which can be elicited by a doctor or primary care worker, are described in more detail in Chapter 5. They include somatic symptoms such as headache or palpitations, excessive anxiety about the baby, sadness and difficulty coping with household tasks. Most mothers are aware they are not their usual selves, but are reluctant to tell others because they fear they will be thought of as incompetent, or regarded as a 'bad mother'.

Postnatal depression is distinguished from the postnatal blues by its greater severity and its longer duration; the postnatal blues being confined to emotional disturbance occuring in the first 2 weeks postpartum.

Puerperal psychosis

A mother with a puerperal psychosis is more obviously disturbed and may have delusions, as well as hallucinations. She may believe she should be punished for being a bad mother, or think she is being followed by the police because of an earlier minor misdeed. Her delusions are often about her baby, which is believed to be dead, deformed or to be evil in some way. Mothers with puerperal psychoses are 'out of touch' with reality and generally lack insight into their disturbed state. Their disturbance of mood is usually obvious to a friend or to a close relative, and psychiatrists are commonly involved at an early stage with the treatment of such mothers, in marked contrast to postnatal depression which is more commonly treated by primary care workers.

Such puerperal psychoses are regarded by a few clinicians as being a specific and distinctive psychiatric diagnosis which is quite separate from other major illnesses such as mania, depressive psychosis or schizophrenia. However, it is more generally agreed that a *depressive* psychosis, perhaps with some atypical features such as perplexity, is the most frequent puerperal psychotic illness; many such depressed mothers remain isolated in their homes and so are less readily recognised as unwell or in need of treatment, because their behaviour is less obviously disturbed.

In developing countries, where there is a greater frequency of physical illnesses, such as parasitic disease or malaria, puerperal psychoses are more likely to have a physical cause and such a mother may then have the typical features of an *organic* psychosis, i.e. clouding of consciousness and disorientation for day, time and place. The greater risk of a neonatal death and of inadequate obstetric care in many developing countries also increase the likelihood of a major mental illness occurring after childbirth. Thus a depressive illness may follow the loss of a baby, or an organic psychosis may be secondary to pelvic infection.

Postnatal blues

The term postnatal blues is restricted to the transitory irritability, weepiness and depression that occur in the first 2 weeks after childbirth, and which do not, by definition, last into the third postnatal week. Although postnatal blues are self-limiting, not uncommonly this mood disturbance may merge into a more prolonged postnatal depressive illness.

RECENT DEVELOPMENTS IN RESEARCH METHODS

There have been two developments in research methodology that have contributed substantially to knowledge about the frequency and the detection of postnatal depression. The first is the development of international criteria for the diagnosis of a depressive illness; one of the difficulties previously encountered, when comparing the frequency of depression following childbirth in different countries, being uncertainty how the word 'depression' was used. The World Health Organization has provided categories of depressive illness, incorporated into the 9th revision of the International Classification of Disease, and there have been attempts to develop other more rigorous ways of classifying depression. Thus the Research Diagnostic Criteria of Spitzer et al (1978) not only consider the presence or absence of depressive symptoms as important in the diagnosis, but also take into account their duration and distress, and whether help was sought. The diagnosis of depressive illness therefore no longer relies on clinical intuition or on a psychoanalytic 'hunch' but on a careful history and information about symptoms of the illness, the distress caused by such symptoms, and their duration.

A second advance in psychiatric research is the use of semi-structured clinical interviews to elicit the psychiatric history in a standardised way. The interviewer proceeds in a way not dissimilar from that of a clinical interview. The success of this form of assessment, however, depends on the interviewer establishing a good rapport with the subject, as well as having controlled empathy. One of the most useful semi-structured interviews is the Standardised Psychiatric Interview Schedule of Goldberg et al (1970). For each psychiatric symptom, e.g. sleep disturbance, depressed mood, anxiety, or psychogenic somatic symptoms, a four-point rating is made according to duration and severity in the previous week. The 'manifest abnormalities' of the patient, e.g. whether a subject appears to be depressed or anxious, has retardation of speech, or psychotic symptoms such as hallucinations or delusions, are also rated using standardised criteria.

The advantage of these interview schedules is that they not only provide ratings for specific symptoms but also allow a formal psychiatric diagnosis to be made. In addition they make it possible to establish rapport with the patient. Information can also be obtained about the past medical and psychiatric history, as well as the social circumstances of the mother.

Self-report scale: development of the Edinburgh Postnatal Depression Scale (PDS)

The third development in research methods of particular relevance to investigating postnatal depression is the use of self-report scales of psychiatric morbidity.

The limitations of existing self-report scales as screening instruments for postnatal depression became apparent to us from our earlier study of 230 women, which used such self-report questionnaires during pregnancy and the puerperium (Cox et al, 1983). The Anxiety and Depression Scale (SAD) of Bedford & Foulds (1978) was chosen initially because it seemed to be appropriate, but was found to have several disadvantages. Not only was the scale insensitive to changes in mood after childbirth, but its validity during pregnancy, as well as in the puerperium, was unsatisfactory.

We found the recommended cut-off of 6 on the total SAD score, if a subject was included in a 'personal illness' category, was inappropriate during pregnancy; of 13 women who scored 6+, only three had a definite psychiatric illness, four had minor symptoms only and six had no evidence of psychiatric morbidity whatsoever.

Another problem was that the scale was unacceptable to some obstetricians, who thought it might *cause* depression, or be upsetting in some other way. An additional item: 'Recently I have been happy and contented' had to be included before it could be used in our study.

Thus, although the SAD had fewer somatic items than most other self-report scales, *any* somatic item was found to be a problem because a morbid somatic symptom rating, such as palpitations, may not indicate an underlying anxiety, but may be caused by the normal physiological changes that occur at childbirth. Insomnia in late pregnancy and after delivery may also be caused by physiological changes or environmental factors and not therefore be associated with a depressed mood.

Limitations of other self-report scales when used to measure psychiatric morbidity in puerperal women have been noted. Thus Nott & Cutts (1982) used the 30-item General Health Questionnaire (GHQ) (Goldberg et al, 1972), which is widely used in community studies of psychiatric morbidity, but found it to have uncertain validity in the puerperium; 45% of the women were high scorers on the GHQ, but only 18% were found to be psychiatric cases at interview.

The Beck Depression Inventory (Beck et al, 1961) is also a commonly used self-report scale to measure depression in community studies, and yet its limitations in the puerperium have been described by O'Hara et al (1983). These authors found that only eight of the 19 subjects who scored 12+ on the Beck scale met clinical Research Diagnostic Criteria for a depressive illness, and of the 23 subjects who scored less than 10, four were nevertheless depressed at interview.

In another study by O'Hara et al (1984), the Beck Depression Scale had other limitations; although significant associations were found between certain cognitive variables before pregnancy and postpartum Beck Depression scores, these associations were *not* upheld when the Research Diagnostic Criteria for postnatal depression based on a clinical interview was the outcome variable. The Beck Depression Scale was also not always acceptable to many field workers and some were reluctant to administer the scale to childbearing women because certain items were regarded as inappropriate. Similar criticisms could also be made of the Zung Depression Scale (Zung, 1965).

Pitt (1968) was the first researcher to devise a more specific self-report measure of postnatal depression. This 24-item scale was administered before and after delivery, and mothers were selected for interview if their scores increased postpartum. This scale was found to be useful in Pitt's study of depression, although its validity as a screening instrument in a busy postnatal clinic was only established for changing, not for absolute scores.

In a thoughtful review of such self-report scales, Williams et al (1980) made the cogent point that all existing scales of psychiatric morbidity should be revalidated for use in community populations where the boundary between psychiatric illness and normality is indistinct, and where 'content' validity and acceptability for use by primary care workers is of critical importance.

Edinburgh Postnatal Depression Scale (PDS)

With these considerations in mind I developed a self-report scale with Jenifer Holden, a psychologist/health visitor and another psychiatrist Ruth Sagovsky. Our aim was to produce a scale to identify postnatal depression in the community which would have satisfactory validity and reliability. Our other requirements were that it should be restricted to identifying postnatal depression, be simple to complete, and acceptable to mothers themselves, as well as to professional health workers.

At the outset we made a detailed analysis of the items on the depression subscale of the Hospital Anxiety and Depression Scale (HAD) (Zigmond & Snaith, 1983), as well as items used in the SAD. The face validity of these items was discussed by two psychiatrists (J.C. and R.S.), a general practitioner (Peter Holland) and Jenifer Holden. In this way a variety of clinical and research experience was used to assess the suitability of each item to detect postnatal depression. We rejected three items: 'I can enjoy a good book or radio or television programme', 'I have lost interest in my appearance', and 'I feel as if I am slowed down', because they lacked face validity for postnatal depression.

We agreed on 21 items, mostly of our own construction, which would include the common symptoms of postnatal depression. These items were then tried out on 50 mothers attending local Health Centres, as well as on women at home. The mothers and health visitors were asked to give their opinion about the appropriateness of items, and in this way we identified items that were ambiguous in meaning, or those which were commonly misconstrued. We retained those items that best discriminated between the depressed and the non-depressed mothers.

Some items that we thought would be particularly useful in the diagnosis of postnatal depression, such as decreased libido, were rejected because they were commonly misunderstood. The item 'I have enjoyed my baby' was also unsatisfactory, since even depressed mothers said they enjoyed their baby. This item was altered to 'I have enjoyed being a mother', because we thought it easier for a depressed mother to admit having less than complete satisfaction with motherhood, than to say she did not enjoy her baby.

From this extensive pilot work the wording of many items was changed, and all were put into the past tense. We then finally agreed on 13 items which we thought were most likely to detect depression in the puerperium (Fig. 1).

In this way we developed a 13-item Postnatal Depression Scale (subsequently abbreviated to a 10-item scale) which consisted of statements describing symptoms of postnatal depression with four possible responses, each graded according to their severity or duration. The mother was asked to underline the response which came closest to how she was feeling in the previous 7 days; each response was scored from 0 to 3 according to severity and a total score derived by adding each of the item scores.

The Postnatal Depression Scale was found to have satisfactory validity when tested against a clinical psychiatric interview carried out on a community sample of women (see Appendix, p 85). Its face validity was satisfactory and it was also acceptable to mothers themselves as well as primary care workers. The PDS as a screening instrument, therefore, was suitable for use by general practitioners, health visitors and midwives to detect postnatal depression in mothers at home, or when they attend the postnatal or baby clinic.

Name: Date:
Address: Age:
                                           Date of Delivery:

As you have recently had a baby, we would like to know how you are feeling now. Please *UNDERLINE* the answer which comes closest to how you have felt IN THE PAST WEEK.

Here is an example, already completed.
I have felt happy:

> Yes, all the time
> <u>Yes, most of the time</u>
> No, not very often
> No, not at all

This would mean: 'I have felt happy most of the time' during the past week. Please complete the other questions in the same way.

IN THE PAST 7 DAYS

1. I have been able to laugh and see the funny side of things

> As much as I always could
> Not quite so much now
> Definitely not so much now
> Not at all

* 2. People upset me so that I felt like slamming doors and banging about

> Yes, often
> Yes, sometimes
> Only occasionally
> Not at all

3. I have looked forward with enjoyment to things:

> As much as I ever did
> Rather less than I used to
> Definitely less than I used to
> Hardly at all

4. I have blamed myself unnecessarily when things went wrong

> Yes, most of the time
> Yes, some of the time
> Not very often
> No, never

5. I have been anxious or worried for no good reason

> No, not at all
> Hardly ever
> Yes, sometimes
> Yes, very often

* 6. I have enjoyed being a mother

> Yes, very much so
> Yes, on the whole
> Rather less than usual
> No, not very much

7. I have felt scared or panicky for no very good reason

> Yes, quite a lot
> Yes, sometimes
> No, not much
> No, not at all

8. Things have been getting on top of me:

> Yes, most of the time I haven't been able to cope at all
> Yes, sometimes I haven't been coping as well as usual
> No, most of the time I have coped quite well
> No, I have been coping as well as ever

9. I have been so unhappy that I have had difficulty sleeping

> Yes, most of the time
> Yes, sometimes
> Not very often
> No, not at all

10. I have felt sad or miserable

> Yes, most of the time
> Yes, quite often
> Not very often
> No, not at all

* 11. I have felt I might lose control and hit someone

> Yes, frequently
> Yes, sometimes
> Only occasionally
> Never

12. I have been so unhappy that I have been crying

> Yes, most of the time
> Yes, quite often
> Only occasionaly
> No, never

13. The thought of harming myself has occured to me:

> Yes, quite often
> Sometimes
> Hardly ever
> Never

---

* = items omitted in the 10-item PDS

Fig. 1 13-Item PDS questionnaire

RESULTS OF HOSPITAL AND COMMUNITY STUDIES

The remaining sections of this chapter describe the results of community as well as hospital based studies of the frequency, symptoms and causes of puerperal mood disorders.

Historical background

The first scientific observations of puerperal mental illness were made during the 19th century by two French psychiatrists. Marcé, in 1858, published a book which contained detailed descriptions of 310 mothers who had a mental illness associated with childbirth, and observed that a particular cluster of psychiatric symptoms was characteristic of mental illnesses in the puerperium. In particular he made the first clinical observation that such mothers were perplexed and disorientated, features usually suggestive of an organic cause for the psychiatric disturbance. Marcé's book has been summarised by Hamilton (1962) and so is now more accessible for English language readers.

In 1845 another French psychiatrist, Esquirol also made pertinent observations about puerperal mental illness, and reported that large numbers of puerperal mothers with 'mild to moderate psychiatric disorder' were cared for at home and 'never recorded'. Despite these astute French observations, however, most subsequent research was of mothers admitted to a psychiatric hospital with florid major puerperal psychoses that required urgent psychiatric management, and only a few studies included mothers who were depressed at home.

Recent studies

One of the most extensive early studies of major puerperal mental illness was carried out by Protheroe (1969), who reviewed the psychiatric case records of puerperal mothers admitted to St Nicholas Hospital in Newscastle upon Tyne between 1927 and 1961. Mothers were included in this study if their mental illness occurred within 6 months following childbirth. One of his most important findings was that these major puerperal mental illnesses had a significant mortality before 1941. Thus of the 52 women admitted between 1927 and 1941, 13 died whilst in hospital. A close temporal relationship was also found between puerperal psychoses and childbirth, a finding later confirmed by Paffenbarger (1964) who found that in 80% the onset of mental illness had occurred within 6 weeks of childbirth. First-time mothers were particularly at risk.

The important question to be answered, however, was whether there was a greater risk of mental illness in puerperal mothers than in mothers who were not childbearing. Pugh et al (1963) investigated this important hypothesis and speculated that, if childbearing had no relationship to psychiatric disorder then no difference in the frequency of psychiatric morbidity between the childbearing mothers and a control group of non-childbearing women, would be found. However the additional risk of a mother being admitted to hospital for the first time with a puerperal psychosis compared with a non-childbearing mother was 0.27 per thousand.

The study that confirmed beyond doubt the increased risk of psychiatric morbidity following childbirth was carried out by Kendell and colleagues (1981) in Edinburgh. These researchers had access to two case registers; a psychiatric register which contained all psychiatric contacts to Edinburgh mental hospitals, and an obstetric case register of all mothers in contact with obstetric services. Using these sources of data 71 240 women, who had recently had a live birth (or stillbirth) in an Edinburgh hospital, were surveyed and the proportion admitted to mental hospital between 1970 and 1977 was established. The time interval before and after childbirth was divided into eight equal 90-day periods. Figure 2 shows their main finding of a striking 16-fold increase in the likelihood of a mother being admitted to a mental hospital 3 months after childbirth compared with the 3 month periods from 1 year before to 1 year after childbirth.

A depressive illness was the most common puerperal mental illness identified in this study, and only one mother had schizophrenia. This low incidence of schizophrenia and also of organic psychoses was in marked contrast with earlier studies in the UK, and with observations in Third World countries (Ebie, 1972; Swift, 1972).

The women admitted to a psychiatric hospital were more likely to have had their first baby, to be unmarried and to have had a caesarean section; findings which confirm popular beliefs that unmarried women having a first baby are more at risk of psychiatric disorder. However when the sub-categories of psychiatric disorder were considered, mothers with a depressive illness were *not* more likely to be single or to be primigravidae.

In a further study by Dean & Kendell (1981), mothers admitted

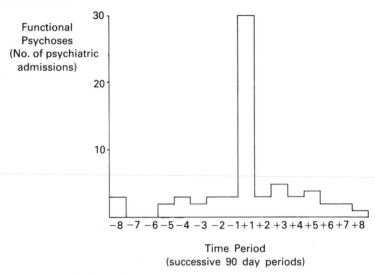

Fig. 2 Temporal relationship between psychiatric admission for functional psychosis and childbirth.

to a mental hospital within 90 days of childbirth were compared with a control group of women admitted with a mental illness that did not follow childbirth. These authors found that the duration of stay in the psychiatric hospital and type of psychiatric treatment did not distinguish between these two groups. The onset of the puerperal mental illness was usually within the first 2 weeks after childbirth; mothers with puerperal mania being more likely to be admitted earlier in the puerperium than a depressed mother.

These studies show that there is indeed a substantial increase in the likelihood of a mother being admitted to a mental hospital after childbirth than at other times, but that the explanation for this increased risk, whether it is due to a lowered threshold for psychiatric referral by the health visitor or general practitioner, is not clarified.

To investigate this matter further, we therefore carried out a prospective community study of postnatal depression which was not restricted to mothers admitted to psychiatric hospital. Instead we studied a sample fully representative of childbearing women in Edinburgh; before describing these results, however, the contributions of other researchers to our understanding of postnatal depression will be outlined.

Postnatal depression

The first community study of post-natal depression was carried out by Brice Pitt in London. He investigated 305 mothers who were attending the antenatal clinics at the London Hospital. To identify those mothers who were depressed after delivery, he designed a 24-item depression rating scale to be completed in the last trimester of pregnancy, and then again 6–8 weeks after delivery. Pitt interviewed those mothers whose score on this scale increased by 6 points between these two occasions, and who were then regarded as being potential depressives. The criteria he used for a depressive illness were as follows:

1. the mother should describe depressive symptoms which had developed since delivery
2. the depressive symptoms should have lasted for at least 2 weeks, be unusual in their intensity and be to some extent socially disabling.

Pitt found that at least 10% were suffering from a marked depressive illness, which was similar in most respects to a neurotic depression. Furthermore if other psychiatric disorders were included, such as anxiety states or obsessive compulsive neuroses, then the frequency of psychiatric morbidity increased yet further to a startling 20%. This study thus provided the first contemporary scientific confirmation of Esquirol's original observation made 100 years earlier that there was indeed a high frequency of untreated postnatal depression amongst mothers living in the community who were 'never recorded' in hospital statistics.

These depressed women were not more likely to have had a forceps delivery, or to be unmarried, or to be older than the women who were not depressed. Mothers with severe postnatal blues however were more at risk of becoming depressed several weeks later, and a previous psychiatric history also increased the risk.

This high prevalence rate of 10% for postnatal depression found by Pitt has been confirmed by most subsequent studies, and is a minimum estimate. A study from general practice by Playfair & Gowers (1981) also found that 10% of mothers were depressed postpartum, whilst in Sweden, Nilsson & Almgren (1970) found a yet higher proportion; 19% of 140 women studied had 'definite signs of psychiatric disturbance' in the puerperium and a further 22% had psychiatric morbidity of lesser severity.

More recently Kumar & Robson (1984), in their study of married primigravidae attending a London teaching hospital, found that 14% were suffering from a depressive neurosis following childbirth. Likewise Watson et al (1984) found 12% of mothers to have a marked affective disorder (predominantly depression) 6 weeks postpartum.

In our own research (Cox et al, 1982) we also carried out a prospective study of postnatal depression and investigated a sample of childbearing mothers fully representative of mothers living in Edinburgh. We carried out detailed assessments of the time of onset as well as the duration of depression that occurred at any time since delivery.

The Standardised Psychiatric Interview, developed by Goldberg for use in community studies of psychiatric morbidity, was administered on four occasions. The first interview (AN1) took place at the mother's first attendance at the antenatal clinic and the second (AN2) was carried out during the last trimester of pregnancy; the third (PN1) occurred within 10 days following childbirth and the fourth (PN2) took place between 3 and 5 months following delivery.

Of the 105 mothers first interviewed at their booking-in clinic, 103 were successfully interviewed 4 months postpartum (PN2). The Standardised Psychiatric Interview allowed the interviewing style to be similar to that of a routine psychiatric interview and good rapport with the mother could be maintained, despite the need to elicit detailed information about defined symptoms. The psychiatric diagnosis was made using the criteria developed by Brice Pitt.

Our main finding, shown in Figure 3, was that 13 (13%) of 103 women had a marked and disabling depressive illness at PN2, 3–5 months postpartum. These mothers had been depressed continuously since delivery and all would have required active treatment by primary care workers. In addition a further 17 (16%) had milder depressions which, though remitted by PN2, were nevertheless unpleasant and had usually lasted for at least 6 weeks. These milder depressions (referred to as depressive 'symptoms' in Figure 3) are distinguished from postnatal blues by their longer duration. If the two categories of postnatal depression (13% depressive illness, 16% depressive symptoms) are combined, then almost one-third (29%) of mothers had been depressed at some time since delivery.

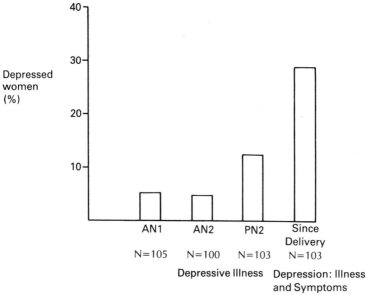

Fig. 3 Depression at AN1, AN2 and PN2.

We could find no association between antenatal obstetric complications or method of delivery and postnatal depression. Furthermore the duration of labour and parity were also unrelated to postnatal mood disturbance. Like Pitt, we could find no evidence that single mothers were more at risk; nor, more surprisingly, were mothers from lower social classes. As in Pitt's study, however, we found a close association between severe blues and postnatal depression; of the 16 mothers with severe postnatal blues, 4 (25%) experienced a prolonged depressive illness that lasted at least until the PN2 interview.

The majority of women with postnatal depression reported having a low mood and said they were 'down in the dumps' or dispirited. This mood disturbance usually started shortly after delivery; some described labile moods and said they were like 'Jekyll and Hyde'. Most had marked sleep disturbance that was readily distinguished from the kind of sleep disturbance caused by a noisy baby, or by the husband's shift work. The self-esteem of the depressed mothers was low and they doubted their ability to cope with household tasks, as well as with their baby. Some mothers were afraid to leave their house because they feared being criticised by others, and most described much unhappiness in their marriage and reported their sexual drive to be markedly reduced. The main reason for this reduced sexual interest was their own lack of libido, seemingly related to the depressed mood rather than to some other factor such as a painful episiotomy or worries about effective contraception. Many depressed mothers also appeared sad and anxious, and some were tearful.

Despite this substantial epidemiological evidence of a high frequency of puerperal depression, it is surprising that this illness is still regarded by some clinicians as trivial and so does not warrant extensive efforts being made to make the diagnosis, or to provide effective treatment. Because such attitudes might diminish the importance attached to training health visitors, midwives and general practitioners in the recognition of postnatal depression, we decided to investigate whether the depressed mothers themselves would accurately recall the duration and intensity of depression when re-interviewed 3 years later (PN3). Our hypothesis was that if non-hospitalised postnatal depression was indeed 'trivial', then it would not be readily recalled by the mothers themselves.

As part of a 3 year follow-up study of the effect of postnatal depression on child development, therefore, we investigated the accuracy of a mother's recall of her earlier puerperal depression (Cox et al, 1984). We re-interviewed 91 of the 103 mothers who had previously taken part in the prospective study just described. These mothers were re-interviewed in their homes by a social worker who did not know whether or not the mother had been depressed following childbirth. The mother was asked whether she recalled being depressed or anxious at any time since childbirth 3 years previously. If such depression was acknowledged, the severity and duration of the depressive symptoms were determined.

Our findings about such 'recalled' depression were quite striking. Of the 92 women interviewed at PN3 17 (20%) said they had been depressed during the 3-4 months after childbirth; the mean duration of depression being 12 weeks. In 7 of 11 women with depressive illness at PN2 the depression had been almost continuous for the first postpartum year. Of the 4 mothers who did not recall having a prolonged depression, but were known to have been depressed, three (subjects 8, 9 and 10) had had a depression following a further pregnancy which had been so severe that they had failed to recall the earlier depression (Fig. 4). The mother's memory was surprisingly accurate, and an 88% agreement was

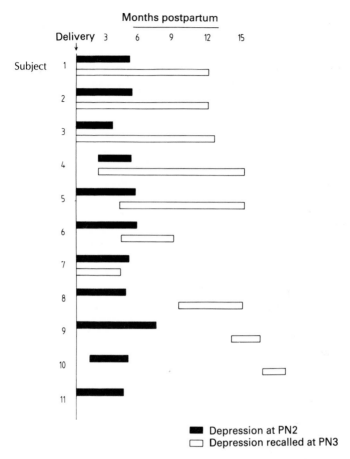

Fig. 4 Agreement between recalled depression (☐) 3 years later and depression observed at PN2 (■)

found between the severity of depression rated in our earlier study and the severity of such depression when recalled 3 years later.

These findings suggest that a puerperal depression, which may not require treatment by a psychiatrist, is nevertheless for the mother a memorable illness, and that its memory may last for several years and influence the attitude to a subsequent pregnancy.

To determine the impact of postnatal depression on the family we then investigated whether the children of depressed mothers would show any more behaviour disturbance than children whose mothers had not been depressed following their birth. With Robert Wrate, Ann Rooney and Philip Thomas we therefore planned to replicate the study of Uddenberg & Englesson (1978) who had found an association between postnatal 'mental disturbance' and a mother's tendency to describe her child in a negative way. The children of mothers who had a puerperal psychiatric disorder in this Swedish study also described their mothers more negatively than children whose mothers had not been depressed.

Our own study however was restricted to assessing only behaviour disturbance in 3-year-old children whose mothers had taken part in the earlier study of postnatal depression (Wrate et al, 1985). We used the Behavioural Screening Questionnaire devised by Naomi Richman (Richman & Graham, 1971) in which the mother is asked a series of questions about aspects of her child's behaviour, and the interviewer rates these behavioural difficulties according to specific rating instructions. The interviewer did not know whether the mother being assessed had had postnatal depression previously.

Our findings again were striking. At first we were reassured that the children of the 11 mothers who had a prolonged previous postnatal depression did not have increased behaviour disturbance, when compared with children of non-depressed mothers. When we examined the subgroup of children whose mothers had shorter depressive episodes postpartum, however, we found that such children *did* have significantly higher scores on the Richman Behavioural Screening Questionnaire than the children of non-depressed mothers. Further analysis of our data was therefore carried out looking for other differences between those mothers with prolonged postnatal depression and those with briefer depressive episodes. We found that mothers with the shorter depressive episodes were those who had had a specific difficulty in mothering and were more likely to be primiparae, to have had difficulty breast-feeding and to have had an early separation from their own mother. Such mothers reported anxiety about their baby and seemed less certain about their own mothering role.

REFERENCES

Beck A T, Ward C H, Mendelson M, Moch J, Erbaugh J 1961 An inventory for measuring depression. Archives of General Psychiatry 4: 53-63
Bedford A, Foulds G 1978 Delusions-symptoms-states. State of Anxiety and Depression (Manual). N.F.E.R. Publishing Company,

Cox J L, Connor Y M, Kendell R E 1982 Prospective study of the Psychiatric Disorders of Childbirth. British Journal of Psychiatry 140:111-117

Cox J L, Connor Y M, Henderson I, McGuire R J, Kendell R E 1983 Prospective study of the psychiatric disorders of childbirth by self-report questionnaire. Journal of Affective Disorders 5:1-7

Cox J L, Rooney, A, Thomas P F, Wrate R W 1984 How accurately do mothers recall postnatal depression? Further data from a 3 year follow-up study. Journal of Psychosomatic Obstetrics and Gynaecology, 3: 185-189

Cox J L, Holden J, Sagovsky R 1985 The detection of postnatal depression by 10-item self report questionnaire: development of the Edinburgh Postnatal Depression Scale EPDS (awaiting publication British Journal of Psychiatry)

Dean C, Kendell R E 1981 The symptomatology of puerperal illness. British Journal of Psychiatry 139: 128-133

Ebie J C 1972 Psychiatric illness in the puerperium among Nigerians. Tropical Geographical Medicine 24: 253-256

Esquirol E 1845 Mental maladies: a treatise on insanities trans. Hunt E K, Lea and Blanchard, Philadelphia

Goldberg D P et al 1972 The detection of psychiatric illness by questionnaire. Maudsley Monograph 21. Oxford University Press, London

Goldberg D P, Cooper B, Eastwood M R, Kedward H B, Shepherd M 1970 A standardised psychiatric interview for use in community surveys. British Journal of Preventive and Social Medicine 24: 18-23

Hamilton J A 1962 Postpartum psychiatric problems. Mosby Harwin, St Louis

Kendell R E, Rennie D, Clark J A, Dean C 1981 The social and obstetric correlates of psychiatric admission in the puerperium. Psychological Medicine 11: 351-359

Kumar R, Robson K 1984 A prospective study of emotional disorders in childbearing women. British Journal of Psychiatry 144: 35-47

Marcé L V 1858 Traite de la folie des femmes enceintes des nouvelles accouches et des nourrices. Bailliére, Paris

Nilssen A, Almgren P E 1970 Paranatal emotional adjustment — a prospective investigation of 165 women. Acta Psychiatrica Scandinavica, Suppl. 220

Nott P N, Cutts, S 1982 Validation of the 30-item General Health Questionnaire in postpartum women. Psychological Medicine 12: 409-413

O'Hara M, Rehm L P, Campbell S B 1983 Postpartum depression: a role for social network and life stress variables. Journal of Nervous and Mental Disease 171:336-341

O'Hara M W, Neunaber D J, Zekoski E M 1984 Prospective study of postpartum depression: prevalence, course and predictive factors. Journal of Abnormal Psychology 93: 158-171

Paffenbarger R S 1964 Picture puzzle of the postpartum psychosis. Journal of Nervous Diseases 13: 161-173

Pitt B 1968 'Atypical' depression following childbirth. British Journal of Psychiatry 114:1325-1335

Playfair H R, Gowers J L 1981 Depression following childbirth — a search for predictive signs. Journal of Royal College of General Practitioners 31:201-208

Protheroe C 1969 Puerperal psychoses: a long-term study. British Journal of Psychiatry 115:9-30

Pugh T F, Jeratt B K, Schmidt W M, Read R B 1963 Rates of mental disease related to childbearing. New England Journal of Medicine 268:1224-1228

Richman N, Graham P J 1971 A Behavioural Screening Questionnaire for use with 3-year-old children: preliminary findings. Journal of Child Psychology 12:5

Spitzer R L, Endicott J, Robins E 1978 Reseach diagnostic criteria. In: Biometrics Research, NY State, Department of Mental Hygiene, New York

Swift C R 1972 Psychosis during the puerperium among Tanzanians. East African Medical Journal 49:651-657

Uddenberg N and Englesson I 1978 Prognosis of post-partum mental disturbance — a prospective study of primiparous women and their 4½ year-old children. Acta Psychiatrica Scandinavica 1958:201-212

Watson J P, Elliott S A, Rugg A J, Brough D I 1984 Psychiatric disorder in pregnancy and the first postnatal year. British Journal of Psychiatry 144:453-462

Williams et al 1980 Case definition and case identification in psychiatric epidemiology: review and assessment. Psychological Medicine 10: 101-114

Wrate R M, Rooney A C, Thomas P F, Cox J L 1985 Postnatal depression and child development: a 3 year follow up study. British Journal of Psychiatry 146:622-627

Zigmond A S, Snaith R P 1983 The Hospital Anxiety and Depression Scale. Acta Psychiatrica Scandinavica 67:361-370

Zung W W K 1965 A self rating depression scale. Archives of General Psychiatry 12:63

4

Causes of postnatal depression

INTRODUCTION

Many health professionals have their own favourite idea about the most likely cause of postnatal depression; some popular explanations, such as progesterone deficiency or the medicalisation of childbirth, are persuasively advocated (see Dalton, 1971). Other popular theories link postnatal depression with the feminist movement, or with the unavailability of parents for support, whilst some suggest that postnatal depression is a product of a Western society and is therefore unlikely to be found in Asia or Africa.

Such explanations are important, however, not only to the extent that they are tenable hypotheses, but also because they partially indicate prevailing attitudes towards childbirth, which in turn influence compliance with treatment and the adequacy of service provision.

The causes of postnatal depression will be discussed by bringing together those explanatory theories that have received substantial support from scientific research, or from established psychodynamic theory.

PSYCHOLOGICAL CONSIDERATIONS

In her useful monograph, Breen (1975) describes childbirth as either a 'hurdle' to be overcome or a 'continuous process' that leads to irreversible physical and psychological change. Breen herself prefers the 'process' theory, because it links the understanding of pregnancy with the process of puberty; both being 'biosocial' events which necessitate the reassessment of personal relationships as well as the acceptance of a new biological role. The young primigravida, for example, has to renegotiate her relationship with her husband as well as with her own mother, and yet in addition must establish an entirely new bond to her baby.

Other psychoanalysts, such as Helene Deutsch (1947), have drawn specific attention to the process of identification that often occurs during childbearing between the mother and her baby, as well as with her own mother. An awareness of these cross-generational links is useful clinically and often helps us to understand a mother's presenting problems.

Thus, a woman with a hostile relationship towards her own mother may find that this identification makes it difficult to be a 'good enough' mother herself. This conflict may then be projected onto the baby who is regarded as unwanted, or even rejected altogether (Fig. 5). Stephen Wolkind and colleagues (1976) found evidence to support these theories and showed that mothers who themselves were deprived of attention in their childhood had greater difficulty accepting their maternal role.

Other support for these theories comes from Nilsson & Almgren's (1970) study in Sweden which showed that postpartum psychiatric disorders were more likely to occur in women with a poor relationship to their own mothers, or in mothers uncertain of their female identity. We also found that women whose own mothers were absent after childbirth usually through earlier death or because of a split family, were more likely to experience severe postnatal blues than women whose own mothers could visit or make contact in some other way.

Other psychological theories of postnatal depression include the 'learned helplessness' theory of Seligman (1975). In this theory depression is thought to result from an inability to avoid unpleasant experiences. The mother believes, for example, that in whatever way she looks after her baby, she will fail in this task and adverse consequences will result from this failure. She is then, according to Seligman, in a state of 'learned helplessness' or depression.

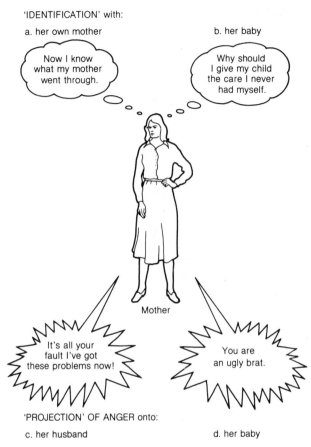

Fig. 5 Identification and projection: common psychological 'defence mechanisms' in the puerperium.

Another recent theory of depression is put forward by Beck (1967), who assumed that a depressed mood was not the primary process in depression, but arises because of the negative way an individual views either herself or the surrounding environment. Thus a mother who has learned always to regard herself as incompetent, has this belief reinforced by difficulties with child-care and so develops a secondary depressed mood. Beck has devised a scheme of cognitive therapy whereby a patient is encouraged first to notice negative thoughts and then to alter and correct them.

These theories assume that such personality attributes are acquired in childhood and that subsequent life stresses, such as childbirth, may provoke depression. Because these explanations for depression are similar to those put forward by mothers themselves, they may lead to useful therapeutic strategies in certain instances.

The possible relationship of personality to puerperal mental illness is also important and has been outlined by Tetlow (1955), who summarised three ways in which personality factors might relate to postnatal depression:

1. The 'Achilles heel' theory—some women have a specific difficulty in mothering or with regard to their sexuality which predisposes them to developing psychiatric disorder, particularly after childbirth.
2. Some mothers are always worriers, and childbirth is therefore just another life event that may cause a mental illness, but there is no particular vulnerability of the personality that specifically relates to childbearing.
3. Any relationship found between personality and puerperal mental illness is entirely coincidental and not likely to occur more frequently than that which could be explained by chance alone. Research evidence, however, is conflicting on this important point, and some authors such as Watson et al (1984) find a relationship between neuroticism scores and postnatal depression, although in our own study no such clear relationship emerged.

SOCIAL CONSIDERATIONS

It is well known that women are more carefully scrutinised by health workers during childbearing months than at almost any other time. The under-utilisers of obstetric services have been studied in detail, and found to come from lower social classes and to have an increased risk of obstetric and psychological complications of childbirth (McKinlay, 1970). Milio (1975) has even suggested their reason for not attending an antenatal clinic is that obstetric services are middle class institutions organised for middle class women and that working class mothers feel alienated from them. However no study has shown a definite relationship between lower social class and postnatal depression, although this association is well established for depression that occurs at other times. Thus in Brown & Harris's study (1978) of depression in Camberwell, working class women were more at risk of depression at any time, and mothers with three or more children under the age of 14 years, and who lacked a confidante, were particularly vulnerable to the impact of life events. Although unmarried women in Camberwell were more at risk of being depressed at any time, studies of postnatal depression have found no such clear relationship with marital status.

Antenatal depression on the other hand in the African and Scottish studies *was* more closely linked to marital status; single, separated or divorced mothers being more at risk of depression prior to childbirth. An illegitimate preganancy was particularly stigmatising in Uganda, because the baby could not then be placed in a family or clan.

No British study has yet investigated the possible relationship between postnatal depression and the place of delivery and these studies are increasingly difficult to carry out because of the rarity of home deliveries. However there was no increased frequency of depression in Africans who delivered in a maternity unit when compared with those who had a home delivery, where traditional birth rituals could more readily be carried out.

The impact of life events, other than the childbirth event, on postnatal depression is now being more carefully evaluated, and Paykel et al (1980) have suggested that childbirth may be a vulnerability factor which enhances the negative impact of another event, such as bereavement or divorce.

BIOLOGICAL FACTORS

The possibility that puerperal depression is caused by biological changes receives substantial support from the literature. Thus Pitt found an association between premenstrual tension and postnatal depression, both of which could be caused by hormonal changes. Further support for the importance of biological factors in the aetiology of postnatal depression comes from studies of patients with manic depressive illness. Thus Reich & Winokur (1970) found a one in three risk of a mother developing a postnatal mental illness if there was a previous history, as well as a family history, of psychiatric disorder and genetic factors are likely to exert their effect on mood through their control of neurochemical processes in the brain, such as releasing neurotransmitters at central brain synapses.

The finding that postnatal blues occur on the fifth postpartum day and that puerperal psychoses also commence at that time would suggest that these two disorders are related to the same initial biological trigger; a major psychosis then may occur in a mother who is vulnerable to mental illness because of a strong genetic loading.

Indirect evidence in support of biological causes comes from other studies which do not find social and obstetric variables to be important predictors of postnatal depression. Thus the popular belief that postnatal depression is more likely to follow an abnormal delivery, toxaemia, or postpartum haemorrhage, is not supported by such studies; although the finding of Kendell et al (1981) that mothers were more likely to be admitted to hospital with a psychiatric illness following caesarean section suggested that such women were at slightly higher risk of puerperal mental illness than mothers who had normal deliveries.

A possible causal synthesis

From this account of possible causal factors of puerperal depression, summarised in Figure 6, it is apparent that the interaction between these biological, psychological and social factors is extremely complex. Thus, although there is no doubt that there is an increased risk of mental illness after childbirth, our knowledge is still limited as to which factors are important in the aetiological chain. The need to consider the impact of life events other than childbirth in the causation of postnatal depression is important; childbirth perhaps being best regarded as a cluster of events, some of which are 'losses' associated with an altered relationship with a partner or with a loss of social role.

An attempt to bring together these various possible causes of postnatal depression arises from considering the work of Schachter & Singer (1962) who investigated the relationship between somatic manifestations of anxiety and the mood actually experienced. Their experiment indicated a model for understanding the interaction between biological and psychological mechanisms underlying mood disturbance. They found that the emotion experienced by

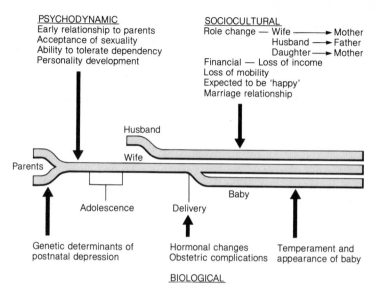

Fig. 6 Possible causal factors in postnatal depression.

an experimental subject, after an injection of adrenaline which caused emotional arousal, was dependent on the surroundings. Thus if the subject was accompanied by a *happy* stooge and an injection of adrenaline administered then he experienced happiness, whereas if a *sad* stooge was placed with the subject prior to the adrenaline injection, he felt unhappy.

These results may provide a template for a consideration of the causes of postnatal depression. Thus the hormonal changes in the first week of the puerperium may not directly determine the mood of the mother, but nevertheless increase the liability to mood disturbance; the mood actually experienced being determined by the social environment, the valencies of specific social relationships and the poignancy of recalled memories from an earlier loss.

It is likely that further progress towards understanding the aetiology of postnatal depression will occur if neurobiological research, which holds one key to knowledge about causation, is carried out in collaboration with social scientists. Furthermore the way the birth 'life event' is rated needs to be reconsidered so that a fuller account is taken of the social and personal meaning of childbirth for the mother herself.

REFERENCES

Beck A T 1967 Depression: clinical, experimental and theoretical aspects. Staples
    Press, London
Breen D 1975 The birth of a first child. Tavistock. London
Brown G W, Harris T 1978 Social origins of depression. Tavistock, London
Dalton K 1971 Prospective study into puerperal depression. British Journal of
    Psychiatry 118: 689−692
Deutsch H 1947 Psychology of women: Motherhood Vol. II. Research Books,
    London
Kendell R E, Rennie D, Clark J A Dean C 1981 The social and obstetric correlates
    of Psychiatric Admission in the Puerperium. Psychological Medicine.
    11: 351−359
McKinlay J B 1970 The new latecomers for antenetal care. British Journal of
    Preventive and Social Medicine 24: 52−57
Milio N 1975 Values, social class and community health services. In: Cox C,
    Mead A (eds) A sociology of medical practice. Collier-Macmillan, London.
    p. 49−61
Nilsson A, Almgren P E 1970 Paranatal emotional adjustment — a prospective
    investigation of 165 women. Acta Psychiatrica Scandinavica, Suppl. 220
Paykel E S, Emms E M, Fletcher J, Ressaby E S 1980 Life events and social support
    in depression. British Journal of Psychiatry 136: 339−346
Reich T, Winokur G 1970 Postpartum psychoses in patients with manic depressive
    disease. Journal of Nervous Diseases 151: 60−68
Schachter S, Singer J E 1962 Cognitive, social and physiological determinants of
    emotional state. Psychology Review 69: 379−99
Seligman M P 1975 Depression, development and death. Freeman, San Francisco
Tetlow C 1955 Psychosis of childbearing. Journal of Mental Science 101: 624
Watson J P, Elliott S A, Rugg A J, Brough D I 1984 Psychiatric disorder in
    pregnancy and the first postnatal year. British Journal of Psychiatry
    144: 453−462
Wolkind S N, Keuk, S, Chaves L P 1976 Childhood experiences and psychosocial
    status in primiparous women: preliminary findings. British Journal of Psychiatry
    128: 391−396

5

Postnatal depression: diagnosis and management

INTRODUCTION

Although it is evident from the research previously discussed that the most common postpartum neurosis is a depressive illness, obsessive-compulsive neuroses, phobic disorders, hysteria, or anxiety neuroses can also follow childbirth and cause much distress.

Thus a mother with agoraphobia, fearful of leaving home or visiting crowded shops, will find childcare tasks particularly difficult and may be unable to go shopping, or to attend a support group or baby clinic. Public transport is avoided because she fears her baby will cry, and that she will be ridiculed by other passengers, and thought to be a bad mother. Agoraphobia can be treated by behaviour therapies, such as desensitisation or flooding; referral to a clinical psychologist is often appropriate.

Obsessive-compulsive neuroses are less common neurotic disorders. Such mothers have great difficulty with childcare because of their irrational need to carry out repetitive rituals, such as hand washing, or checking doors or gas taps a specific number of times. The mother's mind may be preoccupied with warding off intrusive, aggressive or sexual thoughts. The mother may feel ashamed of having these ego-alien thoughts and believe that she may harm her baby or be violent in some other way. However unless these

41

obsessional symptoms are part of a major depressive illness, it is most unlikely that they will be acted on.

Although obsessive-compulsive neuroses can be regarded as a ritualistic defence against unconscious conflict, the most effective treatments are those based on learning theory and include such techniques as 'thought stopping'. In this treatment a mother learns to interrupt such repetitive thoughts at the command of the therapist, or subvocally herself. She may, for example, learn to say 'stop' whenever the obsessional thought arises. Other behavioural therapies include response prevention, in which carrying out the compulsive response is prevented by persuasion, reassurance or encouragement.

One of the most common neurotic disorders is an anxiety neurosis in which the mother's life is dominated by the somatic symptoms of anxiety, such as palpitations, headaches, sweating palms and restlessness, or by the mental anguish caused by the anxiety itself. The anxious mother has great difficulty getting off to sleep because her mind is preoccupied with rounds of worrying thoughts. Such anxiety may develop into a panic attack which is associated with over-breathing and extreme motor restlessness. The mother may for example suddenly leave a family gathering or impulsively run out of the house. Such panic attacks may only occur in specific situations such as a crowded shop, or whilst waiting for a bus. They are then described as phobic anxiety.

The most effective treatments for anxiety neurosis include relaxation techniques, or other forms of anxiety control management. Such mothers may also require psychodynamic psychotherapy, especially if the anxiety is generated by earlier conflicts with parents. This treatment however is labour intensive, and many women do not have the time for this form of therapy.

The reader is referred to the book by Snaith (1981) for a more detailed description of neurotic disorders including hysteria. It is important to emphasise that these neurotic symptoms may occur in a mother with postnatal depression, and then cause additional distress.

POSTNATAL DEPRESSION

Problems of diagnosis

It is a strange irony that although primary care workers regularly visit mothers in the puerperium it is only rarely that postnatal depression is recognised.

There are several reasons for this oversight. Primary care workers may for example have difficulty in deciding whether the mother has 'normal' sadness or whether her low mood is part of a depressive illness. Even if a health visitor is convinced that the mother is depressed the general practitioner may not agree, and may even resent the health visitor making a psychiatric diagnosis at all.

Some health visitors think they will be 'out of their depth with psychiatric patients' and even if they do identify depression, fear they will not know how to carry out effective treatment.

Such problems of diagnosis are further compounded by the mother's reluctance to describe her inner emotional states and her tendency to report only somatic symptoms. This reluctance to say how she feels may be partially due to fear of criticism by the health workers. The mother is apprehensive that she will be told to 'pull herself together', or be ridiculed for making a fuss.

Furthermore a mother with thoughts of self-harm, or who fears that she will harm her baby, is reluctant to describe such ideas to the health visitor because she fears she will be considered a bad mother or may believe the health visitor will take her baby away.

Difficulties for a general practitioner in diagnosing postnatal depression include the short time allowed for an interview. Some depressed mothers are unlikely to consult their general practitioner because they think their problems are too shameful or trivial. The general practitioner may be reluctant to treat postnatal depression because of the advice by drug companies that antidepressants are contraindicated to a mother who is breastfeeding. The general practitioner also has to consider whether a serious physical post-natal complication is present, such as postpartum haemorrhage, infected episiotomy or a breast abscess, and may be deflected from making a psychiatric diagnosis; if the *major* concern is that an organic disorder should not be missed, then unnecessary laboratory investigations may be carried out. Some mothers en-courage their GP to identify a physical rather than a psychiatric illness and report a somatic symptom rather than describe their emotional turmoil.

Another popular belief that militates against postnatal de-pression being detected is the attitude that depression is 'what most women go through'; the mother is then shamed further because of the persistence and distress of her symptoms. Another major disadvantage for the recognition of postnatal depression is that the pharmaceutical industry seems unable to modify the statement that drugs should not be given to a mother who is breastfeeding. There are two psychotropic drugs (lithium and benzodiazepines) which *are* generally contraindicated to a breast-feeding mother but there is no evidence that antidepressants when given in normal dosage cause serious adverse effects on the baby if the mother continues to breastfeed (Beeley, 1986).

One further difficulty in recognising postnatal depression is due to the problem of co-ordinating different community workers. Depression may commence when there is a transfer of responsibility between the midwife and health visitor, so that the health visitor who has taken over the community care of the mother will take time to get to know her, to assess her personality difficulties and determine the relevance of any previous psychiatric history. This mother may feel it is not worth telling the midwife about her personal difficulties because she will have to repeat them to another health worker. The need to maintain continuity of care between health visitor and midwife throughout the antenatal and postnatal period is therefore a most important therapeutic task.

Making the diagnosis

Making the diagnosis is not always as complicated as it may seem at first, and the primary worker by asking certain questions, and listening carefully to the answers, can usually learn to recognise this disorder without too much difficulty.

The health visitor may already be alert to the possibility that the mother is depressed. Thus the depressed mother may have failed to attend a baby clinic, preferring to remain at home to avoid the stress of social interactions, or be out of her house because of her fear that the professional worker will criticise her. A depressed mother may also be excessively preoccupied with her baby and need constant reassurance about feeding. She may worry about the amount of breast milk and not accept any reassurance or explanation that is given. This depressed mother may show excessive concern by having her baby in the bedroom, or by responding too readily to any small movement or cry. A depressed mother may constantly want help with numerous trivial matters about her baby's food or weight, or may consult her general practitioner about a problem with another family member.

These factors should alert the health professional to the possibility of a mother being depressed, and the diagnosis can then be confirmed by a detailed interview eliciting the following main symptoms:

1. Depressed mood

By asking the question 'Are you feeling depressed or sad these days?' it is generally possible to establish whether the mother has a depressed mood, which is one of the hallmarks of a postnatal depressive illness. However it is only rarely that the mother will spontaneously report that she is 'depressed'. Various other synonyms for depression may be used, and the professional worker will need to clarify what mood disturbance is being experienced and then determine its severity and duration.

Most mothers with a moderately severe depressed mood realise there has been a morbid change in their mood state, and may say that they do not feel their usual self. The onset of this depressed mood can usually be dated to 1 or 2 weeks following childbirth, and may merge with the tearfulness of postnatal blues.

The observation of the mother's appearance in the interview, especially her facial expression or weepiness when talking about family relationships may also alert the health worker to the possibility of an underlying depression. More obvious signs of a severe depressive illness, such as the slowing of bodily movements (psychomotor retardation), are only rarely observed.

2. Sleep disturbance

Sleep disturbance is an important symptom of postnatal depression, and all too often the sleep disturbance caused by emotional turmoil is assumed to be brought about by a crying baby or by a noisy husband. Thus only a careful clinical enquiry will allow the health visitor or general practitioner to determine whether the sleeping difficulty (e.g. early morning wakening) is due to depression. Difficulty getting off to sleep, in which a mother lies awake because her mind is preoccupied with worrying thoughts, is another important clue to an underlying depressive illness. A depressed mother may also complain that during the day she feels constantly fatigued, and so goes to bed to avoid company and to rest.

3. Ideas of not coping, self-blame and guilt

A depressive illness may lower a mother's self-esteem, and so further exacerbate feelings of incompetence and guilt. Thus a depressed mother may say she cannot cope with the baby as well as she should be able to, or as well as her own mother did. Her coping ability may indeed be impaired by her low mood, and tasks she previously carried out with rapidity and thoroughness are delayed or not carried out at all. Her guilt and feelings of incompetence are then further exacerbated and a vicious circle of depressive symptomatology is established. Such depressed mothers, however, despite their low self-esteem, may still persist with breastfeeding and appear to be carrying out the routine babycare tasks satisfactorily.

4. Thoughts of self-harm or of harming the baby

It is important to establish whether suicidal thoughts are present and to determine their persistence, and whether or not there are specific suicidal plans. A past history of impulsive behaviour or the presence of a severe depression would indicate that such risks must be taken seriously. Fleeting thoughts of self-harm without specific plans, in the absence of a severe depressive illness, are common and carry a much reduced risk of suicide being attempted.

5. Rejection of the baby

Occasionally there may be an actual physical rejection of the baby, as when a mother refuses to carry out any childcare tasks, an emotional rejection when a mother says she has no feelings towards the baby, is worried that the mother-baby bond is not present, or thinks that the baby belongs to somebody else and does not feel like hers. This last experience is particularly frightening, because the importance of experiencing this mother-baby bond is often emphasised by health educators and by advertisements.

6. Impaired libido

There are many reasons for a reduction of sexual activity in the puerperium, but one of the most common causes is a depressive illness. Other factors include an infected episiotomy, fatigue associated with nightfeeds, role changes in the family and resentment of a husband who is unsympathetic about his wife's problems.

7. Anxiety

Anxiety, as a mood state, is often accompanied by depression and it is wise to assume, until proved otherwise, that any mother who is anxious is also depressed. The somatic symptoms of anxiety, such as headache or palpitations, are also commonly present.

If careful enquiry is made about the presence or absence of these seven symptoms and careful observation made of the mother's facial expression and of other non-verbal communication, the diagnosis of a depressive illness can usually be made without too much difficulty. Thus any mother who has a marked depressed mood, and at least two symptoms present for at least 2 weeks, can be confidently said to have a mild depressive illness, and if more than five symptoms are present, the illness is more major and urgent treatment may then be mandatory.

Screening for postnatal depression

The Edinburgh Postnatal Depression Scale described in Chapter 4 was found to be suitable for use by health visitors and other health professionals as a screening questionnaire at a postnatal clinic; the scale is acceptable to mothers, as well as to professional workers. Most mothers were honest in their responses to the 13 items and were pleased that the questions related to how they were presently feeling. They were relieved that a professional person was taking their emotional problems seriously.

Treatment

Counselling

Most research workers, as well as clinicians familiar with the treatment of postnatal depression, are insistent that one of the most important aspects of treatment is for the professional worker to have a non-judgemental attitude. Indeed this is regarded as crucial if a worthwhile treatment alliance is to be maintained, and if the mother is to collaborate with other forms of medical intervention.

To carry out this form of counselling is not easy, yet depressed mothers readily recognise the benefits of being able to describe their 'unacceptable' thoughts openly to a professional worker. The mother is reassured that the health worker is not reluctant to listen to her bad feelings about her baby, such as that she wishes the baby had not been born, or that she sometimes feels like rejecting the baby.

Jenifer Holden (1985) has devised a most useful way to introduce counselling to health visitors, and the account on pages 53–57 is taken from her notes of guidance, which were developed as part of our investigation of counselling in the treatment of postnatal depression. Ms Holden regards non-directive counselling as being a particularly important style of management in the treatment of postnatal depression. In this counselling the health visitor or other primary care worker is not usually giving direct advice about what the mother should do or how she should cope with her depression but adopts a more listening attitude, which allows the mother to describe 'exactly how she feels'.

This non-directive approach draws considerably on the theoretical work of Carl Rogers (1951) who emphasised three important qualities for the successful therapist:

genuineness
accurate empathy
non-possessive warmth.

It seems likely that counsellors who adopt these attitudes and are not over-involved with the mother but nevertheless empathic, in the sense of putting themselves in another person's shoes, are likely to be successful. It is indeed common for depressed mothers to say that what they wanted at the time of their depression was for the health visitor to understand 'exactly how they felt'. Too early reassurance of the mother that the depression will lift, or minimising the intensity of her emotional distress by saying that she has 'just got postnatal depression' is unlikely to be appropriate.

In our research it has become abundantly clear that these non-directive skills can readily be acquired by health visitors and are generally regarded as helpful clinical skills to master.

Postnatal support groups

One of the most important developments in the prevention and treatment of postnatal depression has been the establishment of self-help support groups, such as the Association for Post Natal Illness and National Childbirth Trust in the UK, and the Pacific Post Partum Support Society in Canada. These groups help by providing supportive peer group assistance which relieves the isolation of many depressed mothers, as well as disseminating knowledge about depression, and indicating where medical treatments can be obtained. These groups function optimally when they are linked with the professional resources of primary care workers such as general practitioners, social workers, health visitors and also with psychiatrists, so that any mother with severe depression who attends group meetings can be identified by health workers and treatment carefully reviewed. Penny Handford (1985), a social worker in Canada, has comprehensively described a postpartum support group and indicates five components of this peer group support which the women find most useful:

1. confidentiality—being able to discuss their depression in a safe setting.
2. counselling—talking to another woman who has been 'through it' has a cathartic effect.
3. focussing upon herself, her needs, thoughts and feelings
4. sharing—discovering that her feelings are similar to those of other women.
5. support—being caring towards others in the group.

Antidepressants

Postnatal depression usually responds to treatment with antidepressant medication. However, because it is commonly believed that these drugs are contraindicated if the mother is breastfeeding, a mother in need of antidepressants may not be prescribed them or they are given in inadequate dosage. To be effective, amitriptyline, for example, should be prescribed at a dose of 100 mg daily and then increased after a few days to 150 mg daily. A mother should be warned of side-effects which include blurred vision, drowsiness, dry mouth, postural hypotension, constipation, and she should also be told that improvement cannot be expected for at least a fortnight.

Other useful antidepressants include the tetracyclic drugs such as Mianserin, which has fewer side-effects and is somewhat safer if taken as an overdose. In certain depressed patients monoamine oxidase inhibitor drugs are useful but require strict dietary prohibitions of tyramine-containing foods, e.g. meat or yeast extracts, Chianti and cheese.

Treatment with antidepressants should be continued until it is certain whether or not there has been a response. The failure of a depressive illness to respond to treatment may be due to the antidepressant drugs being given in inadequate dosage, or to persistent psychological stresses which have not been recognised. A mother who fails to respond to antidepressant medication and counselling should be referred to a psychiatrist; and any mother with strong and persistent suicidal ideas should also be referred or a domiciliary consultation arranged. If there has been a satisfactory response to antidepressant drugs, then it is generally appropriate to continue this medication for a further 3–4 months at least.

Risks of suicide and infanticide

Although health workers are concerned about the risk of suicide and infanticide, these events are extremely rare and are only likely to occur in a woman with an untreated and severe mental illness. Child abuse, which may present as physical assault, is more likely in a woman with a personality disorder and adverse social circumstances than in a mother who is depressed. However, a mother with a depressive illness who *also* has many other problems, such as frequent job changes, several short-lived male relationships, absent family supports, alcoholism or other drug abuse, *is* at greater risk of causing non-accidental injury to her child. The social worker, as well as other primary care workers, must then be closely involved in deciding on the appropriate management. However, to overreact to any expression of dislike of the child, or to a fear that the mother may harm her baby, can be inappropriate and reduce further the mother's self-esteem.

Role of the family in treatment

A depressive illness which occurs in the puerperium when new relationships are being formed, is a threat to family cohesion, because there is usually relief that the baby has been safely born, and an expectation that the mother will soon be able to return to her previous social role. In a Western society it is unfortunate that there are no well-defined norms or 'postpartum taboos' which would define the obligations and constraints of the puerperium, or would sanction a period of inactivity or a reduction of household tasks. In our society the mother's family expect her to return to normal domestic functioning soon after return from hospital, although at that time she may be physically weak and psychologically vulnerable.

The husband also needs considerable reassurance that his depressed wife will get better, and may benefit from explanations as to how a depressive illness can affect a marital relationship. His annoyance that his wife is appearing to reject his baby can be particularly intense.

Postnatal depression may however *result* from an unhappy marriage; the mother's rejection of the baby and her subsequent guilt being linked more closely with her rejection of her husband.

Other family complications may include the mother's own mother becoming overidentified with her daughter, and wishing to take over the care of the baby. Such behaviour can be inappropriately intrusive, exacerbate further the family problems and also reawaken half-forgotten family feuds.

Other children in the family must adjust to a new sibling and realise their mother cannot always give them her attention. In some circumstances the management of postnatal depression will involve this closer examination of family relationships, and marital or family therapy may be the treatment of choice.

The prognosis for postnatal depression is generally good, provided active treatment is maintained by primary care workers fully familiar with the use of physical treatments and counselling. Furthermore, it is vital that co-ordination between different primary care workers is satisfactory. Most depressed mothers respond fully to treatment within 4–6 weeks, although, for some, the depression may last considerably longer.

The mother and health worker can become discouraged by initial lack of response to treatment which may be due to an adverse response to antidepressants, or to persistence of mood lability as the depression lifts. The mother should be told that only gradually will the number of 'good' days outnumber those that are 'bad'.

REFERENCES

Beeley L 1986 Drugs and breast feeding. In: Stirrat G, Beeley L (ed) Clinics in
  obstetrics and gynaecology: Prescribing in pregnancy, W. B. Saunders, London,
  Vol 8, No 2
Hanford P 1985 Postpartum depression: What is it, what helps? The Canadian Nurse
  January, 30–33
Holden J 1985 Counselling by a health visitor in the treatment of postnatal
  depression. M. Phil. Edinburgh University (to be submitted)
Nelson Jones R 1982 The theory and practice of counselling psychology, Holt,
  Rinehart-Winston,
Patterson C H 1974 Relationship counselling and psychotherapy. Harper and Row,
  New York.
Rogers C 1951 Client-centered therapy. Houghton Mifflin, Boston.
Snaith P 1981 Clinical neurosis. Oxford University Press, Oxford

APPENDIX TO CHAPTER 5

COUNSELLING: INSTRUCTIONS TO PRIMARY CARE WORKERS*

1. What is non-directive counselling?

Non-directive counselling is sometimes known as 'Person-Centred' therapy, because this approach locates power in the client, rather than in the counsellor. The major assumption is that by talking through their feelings with a warm and interested, but *non-inter-fering* other person, clients will gradually come to know themselves better, and find solutions to their own problems. The therapist provides a 'nurturing' atmosphere in which the client learns to reorganise her perception of herself and of the world. This is, of course, a gradual process, and is dependent on the establishment of trust.

2. How does counselling differ from health visiting?

It is assumed that health visitors already act as counsellors in many situations. However, as their role is traditionally that of advisors on health matters, being non-directive may involve a change of emphasis. The main difference in comparison with most health visiting is that you are asked *not* to give any direct advice, but rather to help the client work out how *she* feels about things. This can be seen as a passive rather than an active role, and you may find it quite hard at times to avoid 'jumping in' to say what *you* think. Try to remember, though, that your quietly supportive and encouraging presence can be more helpful than the advice you may be eager to offer.

3. What skills will I need for counselling?

Non-directive counselling is a relationship-based approach, which depends more on the level of emotional development of the counsellor than it does on specific techniques. According to Nelson-Jones (1982), counsellors develop their own orientation to counselling, based on their experience of life. The interpersonal

* With kind permission of Jenifer Holden from *Introduction to Counselling Health Visitors (unpublished)*.

skills you already have as a health visitor will be invaluable. Remember, above all, that the client should be 'centre-stage'. You want to create a warm and comforting environment in which she can feel relaxed and trusting, while at the same time maintaining a little formality. How you do this will be a matter of individual personality (yours, hers, and the interaction of both), but the aim is for closeness rather than intimacy.

There are some pointers you might like to think about for getting the atmosphere right. For instance, body language and eye contact are important. It is usually thought best to sit facing each other, but at an angle, to avoid the possibility of intimidating the mother by a direct confrontation. Choose a distance which feels comfortable to you both, perhaps leaning slightly forward, showing interest and inclusiveness. Aim to be attentive but relaxed. Look directly at the mother to show that you are absorbed by what she is telling you, but be sensitive to individual reactions. Depression is a time of avoidance, and some depressed people may find eye contact threatening, rather than reassuring, especially before they know and trust you.

Ideally your voice should inspire confidence and should encourage the mother to relax. For instance, speaking too loudly may seem aggressive, whereas too soft a voice may mean she has to concentrate to hear you, rather than on her thoughts. If you speak too quickly, the client may feel pressurised, but if you speak too slowly, she may think you are bored. Above all, remember that you should only say the minimum that is needed to enable the client to explore her own train of thought.

4. How should I introduce myself in my new role?

First of all, explain to the client why you are there. She will probably be aware that she needs help, and will have been told to expect your visits. Tell her you would like to see her regularly for the next few weeks, and that you will be acting as a counsellor rather than a health visitor. What you actually say is up to you, but you may like to explain that the main reason for your visits is to help her to find out how she feels about things by talking them through. She may expect that you will offer solutions, so you could explain now that although you may not be giving actual advice, you will 'be there' for her. It will help to establish a sense of commitment on both sides if you arrange a regular time for your visits. You should stress that counselling is best done in conditions of privacy, and ask if she can arrange to be on her own when you come. If you have known her for a while, she may find your new role surprising. Explain that you will still be available to answer queries about the baby, but that you want to keep this time specifically for her.

PROBLEMS OF COUNSELLING

What if the client finds it difficult to talk about her feelings?

Most people who are distressed find it a relief to tell someone about it, but they may need encouragement and 'permission' to speak. Quite a useful way of getting things started is to say something like:

'How have things been going this week?'

This is known as an 'open-ended' question, in other words, one which can't be answered with a simple 'Yes' or 'No'. Once the client starts to talk, just listen, showing by your expression that you are interested. If a silence seems to be non-productive, it can be helpful to repeat a little of what she has just said. For instance, she may say something like:

'I sometimes think I'm just stupid'.

You could then say:

'Stupid?'

You aim is to encourage her to continue with a train of thought. If you were to say:

'Oh, I don't think you're stupid at all!'

you (and she) may never find out *why* she thinks this. She may express thoughts or feelings that seem inappropriate to you, but try always to show acceptance of her right to feel the way she does. If you can keep your own ideas to one side, you will give her the chance not only to work out what it is she feels, but gradually to take responsibility for her feelings.

If in doubt, keep quiet!

A companionable silence can not only encourage your client to pursue her own thoughts but it is also a very powerful way of showing that you are accepting and non-judgemental of the content of what she is saying. By keeping quiet you are also keeping yourself and your own views to one side; you are giving her space in which to discover herself and to grow.

Given the right conditions, encouragement and above all, this psychological space, the depressed mother should gradually feel able to start to explore her feelings and perhaps to learn things about herself that she did not suspect. Your role is quietly to help and encourage her to do this, in whatever way seems best and most comfortable to you.

Patterson (1974) has provided a useful description of what counselling is and what it is not. According to this author, there are seven important statements as to what counselling is:

What counselling is

1. Counselling *is* concerned with influencing voluntary behaviour change on the part of the client (client wants to change and seeks counsellor's help).
2. The purpose of counselling is to provide conditions that facilitate voluntary change (conditions such as the individual's right to make choices and to be independent and autonomous).
3. As in all relationships, limits are imposed on the client. (Limits are determined by counselling goals that are in turn influenced by the counsellor's values and philosophy.)
4. Conditions favouring behavioural change are provided through interviews (not all counselling is interviewing, but counselling always *involves* interviewing).
5. Listening is present in counselling, but not all counselling is listening.
6. The counsellor understands clients. (The distinction between the way others understand and the way counsellors understand is qualitative rather than quantitative, and understanding alone does not differentiate counselling from other situations.)
7. Counselling is conducted in privacy, and the discussion is confidential.

What counselling is not

1. The giving of information, though information may be given in counselling.
2. The giving of advice, suggestions and recommendations. (Advice should be recognised as such and not camouflaged as counselling.)
3. Influencing attitudes, beliefs or behaviour by means of persuading, leading or convincing, no matter how indirectly, subtly or painlessly.
4. Influencing behaviour by admonishing, warning, threatening, or compelling without the use of physical force or coercion. (Counselling is not discipline.)
5. Counselling is not interviewing.

Ideally, the depressed mother should come to view you as a person she can trust with her self-doubts, anxieties and problems, even if this involves talking about the negative feelings she has about motherhood and the marital relationship. Sharing such thoughts with someone who is not shocked by them will be a relief, and help her to see herself as less abnormal. Try not to feel despondent if you feel that progress is slow. The full effect of counselling is sometimes only apparent months later. However, the counselling relationship will have spin-offs in itself. Many mothers have the idea that your role is to make sure she is looking after the baby properly. The fact that you have offered yourself as a listening ear may alter the mother's perception of what health visiting is for: to help people towards a positive enjoyment of health.

6

Puerperal psychoses: diagnosis and management

Puerperal psychoses are uncommon psychiatric disorders and follow 2–3 per 1000 live births. Their satisfactory management, however, requires detailed collaboration between obstetricians, psychiatrists, midwives, health visitors and general practitioners, and medical expertise of the highest order. Thus a mother who suddenly develops a postnatal psychotic illness, associated with restlessness, threats of violence and an uncaring attitude towards her baby will cause much distress to the ward staff as well as to other mothers. She may have partial insight into the extent of her difficulties, and be frightened by her awareness that she is behaving out of character, as well as by her destructive thoughts. A patient with puerperal mania on the other hand may enjoy her elated state, and really believe she has supernatural powers or that her baby has a divine mission.

Quite often ward staff are distressed because they are caught up in the mother's delusional systems and thought to be persecutors. One such mother with a paranoid puerperal psychosis became suspicious of the nursing staff and also believed that the paediatrician was planning to harm her baby.

Thus, unlike those mothers with postnatal depression who may remain undetected at home, a mother with a florid puerperal psychosis is usually recognised as being disturbed and in need of help.

Role of the midwife

The midwife's role is particularly important in the early recognition of puerperal psychoses and identifying mothers at high risk. It is her responsibility to ensure that a history of a previous puerperal psychosis or other psychiatric disorder, and a family history of mental illness is obtained at the booking-in clinic, since these are well-established high risk factors for postnatal mental illness.

The midwife, however, has other tasks to carry out in the management of a mother with a puerperal psychosis, in addition to identifying women at risk. She will need to be involved with the ongoing management of a psychotic mother by ensuring that adequate facilities for the mother and baby are available at the psychiatric unit.

A further diagnostic difficulty for midwives as well as psychiatrists, is that this disorder is one end of a continuum of psychiatric morbidity, and careful observation of a mildly disturbed mother in a postnatal ward is therefore necessary. The postnatal blues (emotionalism in the first 2 weeks postpartum), may merge into a postnatal depression, and an untreated postnatal depression develop into a major depressive psychosis.

Another problem of assessment is caused by a psychotic mother with symptoms that could suggest an underlying physical condition. Thus her mood may be extremely labile, she is perplexed and disorientated for time, place and person, and her level of consciousness is also markedly impaired. However, these abnormalities of the mental state may be present even when there is no underlying physical cause for her psychosis.

A midwife, who has correctly observed a mother to be disturbed or to have strange thoughts, may request a psychiatrist to advise about diagnosis and management, but is then dismayed that the patient's mental state becomes normal a few hours later. It is not uncommon for such a mother to be sent home prematurely and then re-admitted a few days later to a mental hospital.

IDENTIFICATION OF PUERPERAL PSYCHOSES

1. Insomnia

This is one of the most important symptoms of a puerperal psychosis and any mother who has sleep disturbance, which cannot be explained by a noisy postnatal ward or by a difficult crying baby, should be observed particularly carefully. If other evidence of disturbed behaviour or of an abnormal mental state emerges, then the early onset of a puerperal psychosis should be considered.

Insomnia may persist throughout the night; typical of a depressive puerperal psychosis however is early morning wakening. Such a mother, who normally sleeps until 7 o'clock in the morning may waken persistently at 3 a.m. when there is no reason to do so. Difficulty getting off to sleep can also occur if she is preoccupied by worrying thoughts. Sleep disturbance can always be readily assessed by any professional worker. Unfortunately it is too readily attributed to environmental causes and the vital chance to recognise a depression is missed.

2. Mood disturbance

The observation of a mother's mood is an important clinical skill for any primary care worker to acquire. This judgement is made by observing the facial expression, as well as by asking directly how she feels in her 'spirits'. In the early stages of a puerperal psychosis lability of mood is particularly characteristic; the depressed mother is distressed by her inability to concentrate on a task, and perplexed that she is unable to think clearly about child care. She may be abrupt or careless in handling the baby, or in the way she carries out breastfeeding. Her disturbed mood makes it difficult to relate to her baby in a contented way.

3. Unusual behaviour

Behaviour that is out of keeping with the mother's usual personality or with the demands of the postnatal ward routine may be the early sign of a puerperal psychosis. Excessive restlessness, for example pacing up and down the corridor, climbing in and out of bed, or asking staff questions about trivial matters, holding the baby in some strange way, or refusing to care for the baby because she fears harm may come to it, may all be early signs of a major puerperal mental illness. Occasionally extreme forms of excitement occur, as when the mother rushes out of the room in response to a hallucinatory voice or because of some imagined persecutors.

4. Unusual beliefs

Most mothers with a puerperal psychosis have delusions, and these may include the baby, which is believed to be damaged, to have destructive powers or even to be dead. Delusions of guilt are common, for example, that she is a bad mother, or has carried out a minor misdemeanour in the past for which she should be punished. The ward staff are often included in these persecutory beliefs and may be thought to be in secret communication with the police. In a case of manic psychosis the mother may believe that she has special powers, or is a special person, such as a saint or a world leader. She may then handle her baby in a casual or otherwise inappropriate way.

Although it is not difficult to diagnose a major puerperal illness once it has become florid, the diagnosis is more difficult in the early stages of the illness. Midwives and obstetricians however can be helped in this task by talking to the husband to determine what is the mother's normal personality, which may contrast with her present behaviour.

Assessing suicidal risk

A mother with a puerperal psychosis may have strong suicidal thoughts. She may believe that she is a bad person who deserves to die as a punishment for her previous misdeeds, or believe that others would be happy if she died, or that her baby would be better cared for by another person. She may even believe that her baby would be happier if it were not alive, and this can result in infanticide.

Any mother who expresses persistent suicidal or infanticidal thoughts, especially if they occur in the setting of an incipient psychosis or in a mother who is known to be at high risk of a puerperal psychosis, should be carefully observed and psychiatric consultation arranged.

It is clear that whilst primary care workers are important in the early detection of the disorder, psychiatrists are usually involved in the management and treatment of these disturbed mothers. It is an advantage therefore if the psychiatrist can assess the mother on the postnatal ward, or at home, and be involved in the decision to admit the mother to a psychiatric hospital. It is usually possible for the mother to be admitted voluntarily to hospital, although compulsory admission, using the powers of the Mental Health Act, is sometimes needed.

Whether the mother is admitted to a general psychiatric unit, or to a mother and baby unit will depend on what local facilities are available. It is important however that obstetricians, hospital and community midwives, general practitioners and health visitors remain in detailed contact with the mother and her baby during *any* subsequent psychiatric treatment. Close co-operation with paediatricians is also necessary, as there is a risk that a psychiatric team will be more concerned with the mother's psychiatric diagnosis than with other aspects of management, such as feeding problems, so that the baby's physical health may be overlooked.

MOTHER AND BABY UNITS

An account of the mother and baby unit in Manchester is provided by Margison & Brockington (1982) who describe a series of 245 mothers and babies admitted over the last 4 years. This unit was purpose-built with adequate observation arrangements and a nursery; it was staffed by nursery nurses as well as psychiatric nurses, psychiatrists and other health professionals.

However, most regions do not have a purpose-built mother and baby unit and have to share a facility with a general psychiatry ward. The advantages of a mother and baby unit are nevertheless considerable and include the following:

1. Avoids a physical separation of mother and baby, so allowing careful scrutiny of the mother's relationship with her baby; specific assistance can be given if a mother requires psychological support or education about how to look after her baby. In this way her own self-esteem is maintained.
2. Allows the urgent inpatient treatment of a mother who otherwise might have refused help because hospitalisation would mean she was separated from her baby.
3. For single mothers, or those with inadequate social supports to care for the baby, psychiatric treatment can be undertaken urgently without the baby being placed in a foster home.

The organisation of such a mother and baby unit is complex; the anxiety of staff about the safety of the baby may be considerable.

Thus although no case of infanticide was reported by Margison & Brockington, three babies were harmed. The risk of a baby being harmed by another psychotic mother has also to be considered. A patient who had been admitted to a general psychiatry ward with a puerperal psychosis, described how she had regarded another baby on the ward as having evil powers, and at one time she had the intention of harming this baby. This risk of harm to a baby from another psychotic patient is increased if the mother and baby facility is part of a general psychiatry ward and if observational facilities are limited. The minimum requirement of such a facility would therefore be two adjacent lockable rooms, one of which can be used as a nursery. The need to prevent access of other patients to the baby is vital and the feasibility of direct observation by the nurses of the mother with her baby must be carefully assessed. A very disturbed mother, for example, may need to have constant observation by a nurse at all times. Nursing staff levels must be adequate to allow this observation to take place.

The social worker has a particular responsibility to ensure that the baby is in 'a place of safety', and will therefore need to consider the availability of psychiatric nurses to ensure adequate observation, the presence of nursery nurses with specific skills to care for the baby, the adequacy of contact with paediatricians to identify physical abnormalities of the baby, and the risk to the baby from another disturbed mother.

In some units the mother has legal responsibility for her baby and this matter must be clarified with the hospital administration, and a decision made as to whether the baby is a patient or has similar status to a visiting relative.

The decision to admit a mother and baby to a psychiatric hospital is never easy and is especially difficult when the decision involves an intervention in a complex family relationship. Considerable time therefore needs to be given to explain to the husband the nature of his wife's disturbance, and the reasons why he has to be separated from his wife and also from his own child.

Admission of the mother to a psychiatric unit even without the baby may be essential if there is a clear risk of the mother harming her baby at home, or if there is a serious threat of suicide. In some circumstances it may be wise to admit the mother so that her behaviour, and the content of her delusions, can be assessed and the possible risk to the child from the mother's disturbed mental state evaluated.

Margaret Oates (1985) in Nottingham has developed an intensive community service for the domiciliary treatment of mothers with puerperal psychosis, which may be a satisfactory alternative to a more costly mother and baby unit. This service however depends on the commitment of community psychiatric nurses and of psychiatrists and on their constant availability for this most demanding domiciliary psychiatry.

There is no evaluation as yet of a day hospital in the management of women with puerperal psychoses although such an arrangement might provide adequate hospital resources without the need to develop a specific mother and baby inpatient unit.

MANAGEMENT OF PUERPERAL PSYCHOSES

The initial clinical task for the psychiatric team is to make a full assessment of the mother's mental state, and her physical condition. A detailed interview with a relative will also help in making an accurate diagnosis. Particular attention will need to be given to the past psychiatric history, more especially if there has been a previous puerperal psychosis, since this may give some clue to the nature of the present disturbance. Thus a mother who has had a previous manic or depressive illness, will be more likely to suffer from this disorder in the puerperium.

Electroconvulsive therapy in the treatment of puerperal psychoses has been shown to be particularly effective and is especially indicated in a mother with a severe depressive psychosis who is a risk to herself or others, and for whom it would be unwise to wait 2 to 3 weeks to establish whether antidepressant drugs will be effective.

A mother with puerperal mania may cause much disruption to the postnatal ward, as well as to a psychiatric unit. Fortunately this illness usually responds to treatment with Haloperidol or lithium carbonate. Lithium carbonate should also be considered as prophylaxis against further depressive or manic episodes; although particular care has to be taken if there is a strong likelihood that the mother will become pregnant again. If the mother thinks she is pregnant whilst taking lithium, then the drug must be immediately withdrawn.

Most mothers with puerperal psychoses respond promptly to

treatment and although a relapse can occur, the mother's condition is usually substantially improved within 5–6 weeks.

At the assessment stage it may also be important to make a psychodynamic assessment of the mother's difficulties, and to take account of the part played in the aetiology of the illness by her personality, her relationship to her own mother, and the quality of the marital relationship. These factors may not only partially explain the content of the mother's delusions or the reason for her rejecting the baby, but may also suggest what forms of psychotherapy may be necessary. A mother whose puerperal depressive illness is partly related to unresolved feelings about her mother's death, for example, or whose rejection of her baby is linked to her anger towards her husband, may be helped by group or individual psychotherapy.

In addition to psychodynamic psychotherapy, behaviour therapy to encourage the mother to relearn her mothering skills is also important. These methods have been developed successfully in Manchester by Brierley who has used modelling techniques, in which the therapist shows the mother how childcare tasks are carried out, and rewards her for success in developing these skills.

Nursing an impaired mother-infant relationship in puerperal depression has been described by Scott (1984) who suggests that the health worker should answer the question 'What does this baby mean to this mother?' and try to understand how the mother meets the needs of her baby. The importance of the nursing role in this task is correctly emphasised because this assessment requires the constant observation of day-to-day interactions of the mother and baby.

Most mothers with a major puerperal psychosis which requires treatment in a psychiatric hospital are unable to continue breastfeeding, not only because medications (such as lithium or diazepam) are excreted in breastmilk but also because the mother needs rest; and may need to be relieved of feeling that she is personally responsible for her baby's welfare.

The arrangements for discharge from a psychiatric unit to the community necessitate close co-ordination with the primary care workers. The general practitioner needs to be fully informed of the diagnosis and of the drug regime when the patient is discharged. The community health visitor and community psychiatric nurse, who may also have visited the mother in hospital, should be fully briefed about the psychiatric illness, its prognosis and the need for further outpatient treatment.

The health visitor therefore should be familiar with the side-effects of psychotropic drugs, such as phenothiazines and tricyclic antidepressants. The community psychiatric nurse will also be particularly important and can combine her psychiatric skills with those of the health visitor and general practitioner.

The mother and her family can be reassured that recovery from an acute illness is usually complete within 6–8 weeks. However, they should be warned that the risk of a further puerperal psychotic illness following a subsequent pregnancy can be as high as one in five. This risk is particularly great if there is a family history of psychiatric disorder and a previous puerperal psychosis. It is also important that detailed advice is given to the patient about contraception, and it is usually wise to discourage the mother from having another child within a 2-year period.

REFERENCES

Margison F, Brockington I 1982 Psychiatric mother and baby units. In: Brockington I, Kumar R (eds) Motherhood and mental illness. Academic Press,
Oates M 1985 Personal communication
Scott D 1984 Nursing the impaired mother-infant relationship in puerperal depression. The Australian Journal of Advanced Nursing I: 50–56

7

Postnatal blues

The postnatal 'blues' (emotionalism of the first 2 weeks post-partum) have been described for several decades, but it is only in recent years that improved research methods have provided a scientific basis for the further understanding of earlier clinical observations, as well as indicating possible causal factors.

One of the first studies of the postnatal 'blues' was carried out by Robin (1962), who interviewed 25 women in a lying-in ward on or about the ninth postpartum day, and found that 19 (76%) had experienced feelings of depression on at least 1 day after childbirth. He also noted that 16 complained of emotional lability, and that some 'cried at nothing', 'laughed at nothing' or were 'up and down'. Yalom et al (1968), interviewed 39 mothers in hospital six times during the first 3 days after delivery and also telephoned each woman daily for the next 7 days. They found that two-thirds of such mothers had one episode of weeping during this period.

In a study by Pitt (1972) 50 of the 100 women interviewed between the seventh and tenth day postpartum had spells of tearfulness and depression. Mild confusion was found in 23 and consisted of impaired concentration, memory and learning, and Pitt therefore argues that the syndrome is organically determined.

More recent studies from Edinburgh (Kendell et al, 1981) used 10 cm visual analogue scales to measure depression, anxiety, tears, irritability, lability of mood and happiness for the first 21 days postpartum and also investigated the possible relationship between postnatal blues and postnatal depression. The results showed that maximum depression and tearfulness did indeed usually occur on the fifth day postpartum and were not related to the day of discharge from hospital or whether or not the mother was breastfeeding. Our earlier study of postnatal depression had shown that one-quarter of mothers with severe postnatal blues subsequently developed postnatal depression.

In a more recent study, the daily mood ratings of women who were in hospital for a full 10 days after a caesarean section were compared with a control group who had an elective hysterectomy (Kendell et al 1984). In this study we hoped to establish whether the day 5 peak still occurred in women who remained in hospital for 10 days, and to determine whether the blues might occur following *any* lower abdominal operation. Our results, showed that no trace of a fifth day depression followed the hysterectomy, and that the peak of emotionalism was still identifiable on day 5 in the caesarean group.

These findings suggest that fifth day emotionalism is indeed specific to childbirth and not likely to be caused by the mother's excitement about leaving hospital or to be a non-specific reaction to a lower abdominal operation. We also found that those mothers who were most likely to have the blues were those with high neuroticism scores on the Eysenck Personality Inventory, and so may possibly have heightened autonomic responsiveness.

Biological research into the causes of postnatal blues has produced a variety of results. Some authors, such as Ballinger et al (1979), found increased levels of urinary cyclic-AMP in mothers with emotional disturbance on day 3, while Coppen et at (1973) found reduced levels of tryptophan.

Other researchers such as Peters & Elliot (1984) in Oxford found evidence that sex hormones may have an effect on monoamine receptors in the brain which may control the release of noradrenaline—the transmitter substance believed to be related to maintaining normal mood states. As with the other studies cited, 'however' their data about brain function are indirect.

These diverse findings illustrate the methodological problem that the blues occur when numerous biological changes are taking place so that an association found between a biological change and a mood state cannot necessarily be regarded as a causal relationship.

One of the most popular theories advocated firmly by Dalton (1971) is that the postnatal blues are caused by a deficiency of progesterone. But although this explanation is a tenable hypothesis, it has not yet been adequately tested scientifically. We are at present investigating in a double-blind control study, whether dydrogesterone, a derivative of progesterone taken by mouth, has any effect on reducing the severity of postnatal blues.

The challenge for research into postnatal blues is not however solely to find the cause of these transitory mood disturbances, but to provide clues to the aetiology of postnatal depression and the puerperal psychoses.

MANAGEMENT

The assessment of postnatal blues can be difficult because the midwife and obstetrician will need to distinguish those mothers for whom the blues are only a transitory emotional state, from mothers who may be developing postnatal depression, or even a psychosis.

Particular attention should therefore be given to those mothers with severe blues who are known to be at increased risk of postnatal depression because of a history of psychiatric disorder, or a strong family history of mental illness. Such mothers should not be discharged home in an aroused emotional state, but kept in hospital to ensure that their mood has not deteriorated. If they insist on going home it is important that primary care workers are informed that they are likely to become depressed so that additional domiciliary care and early treatment can be initiated if a serious psychiatric disorder develops.

It is beneficial if the midwife listens carefully to what the mother is worried about, and allows her to express irritation with the family, the baby or with the staff. It is unhelpful to dismiss such a mother's distress as 'just the blues', because this trivialises a painful emotional disturbance; to respond to such a mother by being irritated or 'arguing back', is also not therapeutic.

Assistance with medical problems such as cracked nipples, painful episiotomy, urinary or bowel problems is appropriate, and showing understanding of marital problems, and an unwanted or an ill baby is reassuring. Sedative drugs are rarely helpful, unless the mother is excessively anxious.

POSTPARTUM MOOD DISORDER: SUMMARY

Table 1 summarises many of these clinical aspects of the treatment of puerperal psychoses, postnatal depression and postnatal blues. It is clear that the main responsibility for the early recognition of puerperal psychoses, the diagnosis and treatment of postnatal depression, and alleviating the distress of postnatal blues lies with the community-based professional health workers, and that the psychiatrist may only be involved as an educator, or with the treatment of mothers who require psychiatric admission.

It is my experience that health visitors and community midwives cannot leave the task of diagnosis only to the general practitioner,

Table 1 Spectrum of mood disturbance in puerperium

	Postnatal blues	Puerperal depression	Puerperal Psychoses
Frequency	50–70%	10–15%	0·2% affective psychosis – common schizophrenia organic psychoses } rare
Peak time of onset	4–5 days after childbirth	2–3 weeks after childbirth	2–3 weeks after childbirth
Duration	usually 2–3 days	4–6 weeks if treated up to 1 year if untreated	6–12 weeks
	severe 'blues' may →	postnatal → depression	affective psychosis
Professional first contact	midwife (hospital), obstetrician	midwife (community), health visitor, general practitioner	midwife health visitor, general practitioner, psychiatrist (rare)
Psychiatric referral	virtually never	unusual	common — especially if marked behaviour disturbance
Possible treatments	nil: but observation if severe	counselling, antidepressants	admit to mother & baby unit; phenothiazines; lithium; ECT; counselling; advice about pregnancy

and should be encouraged to take full advantage of their right of entry to a mother's home to detect puerperal mental illness, which otherwise might be unrecognised.

If the community-based worker is already aware of the frequency of puerperal mental illness, is on the look-out for mothers who may present their psychiatric problems in unusual ways, and can ask appropriate questions to elicit symptoms, then more mothers with puerperal mental illness would be identified. This diagnostic task can be assisted by using screening questionnaires, but these are not a substitute for a clinical assessment by a professional worker.

REFERENCES

Ballinger C B, Buckley D E, Naylor G J, Stansfield D A 1979 Emotional disturbance following childbirth and the excretion of cyclic AMP. Psychological Medicine 9: 293–300
Coppen A, Eccleston D, Peet M 1973 Total and free tryptophan concentration in the plasma of depressed patients. Lancet ii: 1415–1416
Dalton K 1971 Prospective study of puerperal depression. British Journal of Psychiatry 118: 689–692
Kendell R E, McGuire R J, Connor Y, Cox J L 1981 Mood changes in the first three weeks after childbirth. Journal of Affective Disorders 3: 317–326
Kendell R E, Mackenzie W E, West C, McGuire R J, Cox J L 1984 Day-to-day mood changes after chilbirth: further data. British Journal of Psychiatry 145: 620–625
Peters J R, Elliott J M 1984 Quoted in MRC News, December
Pitt B 1973 Maternity blues. British Journal of Psychiatry 122: 431–435
Robin A A 1962 Psychological changes of normal parturition. Psychiatric Quarterly 36: 129–150
Yalom I D, Lunke D T, Moos R H, Hamburg D A 1965 Postpartum blues syndrome. Archives of General Psychiatry 18: 16–27

8

Prevention

As the personal and social consequences of postnatal depression can be daunting, it would be desirable if this disorder could be prevented by early intervention, or if mothers known to be at high risk could be identified during pregnancy. However, with the exception of mothers who have had a previous postnatal depression or other psychiatric illness, there are few factors that will allow the confident identification of mothers who will become depressed in the puerperium. Thus, although many studies report an association between postnatal depression on the one hand and antenatal psychiatric disturbances, the mother's personality and mental problems on the other, these associations, though statistically significant, are not necessarily useful in clinical practice, since many mothers with these characteristics do not become depressed after childbirth.

The prevention of postnatal depression is considered under three headings:

- Primary prevention — reducing the risk that a mother will develop postnatal depression
- Secondary prevention — making an early diagnosis and then commencing treatment
- Tertiary prevention — reducing the effects of established depression on the family, and on the attitude towards subsequent pregnancies.

PRIMARY PREVENTION

Primary prevention may include the optimum use of drugs, as well as preventive counselling.

Drugs may be used to reduce the likelihood of postnatal occurring in mothers with a definite past history of puerperal depression, or with a family history of manic-depressive illness. In such women an antidepressant, such as amitriptyline, could be prescribed during the third trimester of pregnancy and continued to the puerperium. A pregnant mother with schizophrenia may benefit from a tranquilliser (e.g. thioridazine) being prescribed during the last trimester of pregnancy and after childbirth, to reduce the risk of relapse in the puerperium.

It is not known whether progesterone, given after childbirth to women who are at high risk of postnatal depression, is successful in reducing the likelihood of this illness occurring, and it is an urgent task for studies to be undertaken to determine whether or not hormone prophylaxis is effective.

A mother who has a previous history of manic or depressive illnesses may benefit from prophylactic use of lithium carbonate. However, the control of the serum lithium levels is difficult during the childbearing months, and immediately following delivery because of changes in renal function and electrolyte balance. Lithium is contraindicated if a mother is breastfeeding.

Education of all mothers attending antenatal parentcraft classes may reduce the likelihood of postnatal depression occurring in two main ways:

a. By encouraging the mother to avoid other stressful life events in the puerperium, such as a housemove or change of job;

b. By explaining that there is a likelihood that a mother will experience postnatal blues, or become depressed after childbirth. This topic should not be avoided because it is thought to upset a mother. Most mothers welcome such information and value being informed where to obtain help if they become depressed. Fathers also appreciate being told about the presentation of postnatal depression, and welcome advice about how they can help or manage their own anxiety.

The avoidance of the topic of postnatal depression in antenatal education for fear of upsetting mothers, or of inducing psychiatric disturbance, or 'meddling in psychiatry', is more likely to reflect the attitude of the tutor than the anxieties of the mother. Studies are however needed to demonstrate what attitude changes do occur following antenatal education about puerperal mood disorder. My own experience is that mothers welcome such basic information about puerperal psychiatric disorder, and are relieved to have this information rather than troubled by it. It may be appropriate to give this information to mothers in the postnatal ward; at that time she may be more receptive to these ideas than before delivery.

Some antenatal clinics find that the booklets published by the Association for Postnatal Illness on the Baby Blues and Postnatal Depression provide a coherent account of these emotional states. These leaflets give brief answers to questions the mother commonly asks.

What are the baby blues?
What causes the baby blues?
How will I feel if I get the blues?
How long do the baby blues last?
What is the difference between the baby blues and postnatal depression?
What should I do if I think I have postnatal depression?
Will I get better?
Where can I get help?
Can I help myself?

Another leaflet provides an account of the symptoms of postnatal depression and emphasises that one common symptom of depression is a loss of interest in sex. It contains useful information about how a family can help a depressed mother by ensuring that she is receiving treatment, giving reassurance that the illness is a temporary one, and emphasising that help and support from friends assists recovery. The relatives are advised not to chivvy a mother 'out of her depression'. It is suggested that they should treat her as if she had a physical illness. The family is also urged to assist with household tasks, but when the mother recovers she should be allowed to resume household responsibilities. The depressed mother should be reassured that she will get better, and discouraged from regarding her depression as a sign of weakness.

It is recommended that support for the depressed mother who is reluctant to be left alone could be provided by a rota of helpers. The mother is encouraged to take as much rest as she can, not to go on a strict diet or to have long periods without food and to avoid situations or places which upset her. The booklet concludes by describing the sort of additional help that is available from the National Childbirth Trust, the Meet-a-Mum Association and the telephone counselling offered by the Association for Postnatal Illness.

Education of health professionals

The need for sustained education for professionals involved in the care of childbearing women about motherhood and mental illness cannot be overemphasised. As Oates (1985) has pointed out, at present there is only a requirement of 2 hours teaching for midwives on 'human relationship's and 'the emotional impact on the child'. Yet the response of tutors as well as students to teaching on these topics is perceptive and enthusiastic and the need for such teaching is increasingly being recognised. Margaret Oates has described the aims and objectives of a course entitled 'Education for Care' under eight headings:

1. To increase the sensitivity and perception of the midwife to the mother's emotional changes and emotional needs during pregnancy and the puerperium.
2. To increase the awareness of socio-cultural factors and variation in family life and child-rearing patterns, not only within the majority society, but also in ethnic minority groups.
3. To help the midwife understand and identify those risk factors in individuals and vulnerable populations which can be identified during antenatal care, to enable the midwife to engage in preventative work with women who are more likely to develop emotional disturbances in the puerperium.
4. To help the midwife identify and diagnose in broad terms mental illness in the puerperium and her role in the management of these conditions.
5. To help the midwife to deploy existing resources in antenatal care and postnatal care more effectively.
6. To help the midwife more effectively use parentcraft and antenatal classes.
7. To help the midwife critically evaluate current practices and see areas where improvement might be possible.
8. To increase the awareness of the midwife of the normal process of grief and its problems, particularly in relation to perinatal death and the birth of a handicapped child.

16 hours of this teaching is given by members of the Postnatal Mental Illness Service, and a further 10 hours by midwifery tutors.

SECONDARY PREVENTION

From the foregoing account it is clear that primary prevention of postnatal depression, by reducing the likelihood of it occurring, is difficult to achieve. It is therefore important that the early detection of depression in the puerperium is carried out as effectively as possible, since this is the best way to prevent the adverse consequences of an untreated postnatal depressive illness. A mother who has severe postnatal blues should be closely observed by community workers, and early treatment for depression given if her low mood continues.

In the first days of postnatal depression, the moods are often labile, so that the health visitor, midwife or general practitioner should not too readily he reassured by an apparent improvement, and should therefore continue to observe the mother for several weeks. The postnatal depression scale (PDS) is particularly useful for primary care workers when visiting mothers at home, and will detect many mothers who are depressed. The scale can be used to alert primary care workers to those mothers who require more careful clinical assessment and so enable secondary prevention to be achieved.

Once a depressed mother has been identified, further treatment should be undertaken by the general practitioner in close collaboration with the health visitor, community psychiatric nurse or community midwife. Mothers who are found to have a severe depressive psychosis may then be referred directly to a psychiatrist.

TERTIARY PREVENTION

Postnatal depression, especially if it is prolonged and untreated, may seriously disrupt a marriage and is also clearly remembered by mothers 3 years later (Cox et al, 1984). In some instances the mother says that she would not want to go through with 'that' again. It is fortunate however that the 3-year-old children of mothers with a severe postnatal depression did not have more behavioural disturbance than children whose mothers were not depressed in the puerperium, although a weak association was found between *brief* postnatal depressive episodes and mild behavioural disturbance in the child (Wrate et al, 1985).

Adverse family sequelae of depression are reduced if the parents are given an explanation of how postnatal depression may reduce libido, or increase irritability. The mother and her husband should be advised about the need for adequate contraception; family therapy may also be necessary when adverse attitudes have developed during the illness.

REFERENCES

Cox J L, Rooney A, Thomas P F, Wrate R 1984 How accurately do mothers recall postnatal depression? Further data from a 3 year follow-up study. Journal of Psychosomatic Obstetrics and Gynaecology 3: 185–189
Oates M 1985 Education for care. Unpublished
Wrate R W, Rooney A C, Thomas P F, Cox J L 1985 Postnatal depression and child development: a 3 year follow-up study. British Journal of Psychiatry 146, 622–627

9

Conclusions

Throughout this book it has been emphasised that the diagnosis and treatment of postnatal depression depend to a large extent on persistent and detailed collaboration between the various primary care workers in the community, and hospital-based specialists. At present such co-operation does not always exist, and although puerperal women are regularly assessed, postnatal depression, one of the most disabling postnatal complications, is rarely diagnosed and treated.

It is to be hoped that this book will have encouraged such primary care workers, as well as obstetricians and psychiatrists, to identify postnatal depression more accurately and to undertake appropriate treatments. Mothers themselves increasingly recognise the importance of this disorder, and are alerting the medical profession to the problems caused by depression at this time. The Association for Post-Natal Illness, provides a counselling phone-in service for mothers, and is particularly effective when backed up by adequate medical support.

Fathers also use this support facility, and one father recently explained how relieved he was that his wife's difficulties were immediately understood and recognised by the counsellor. His wife was told how to obtain appropriate treatment for her depressive illness. Such organisations have an important role in promoting research.

It is also encouraging that there is evidence of a growing interest amongst psychiatrists in the puerperal psychoses as well as in the puerperal neuroses. One task of a psychiatrist is to provide education for primary health workers; the psychiatrist may however need to obtain experience of postnatal depression in the community for such teaching to be successful.

The Marcé Society for furthering the understanding, prevention and treatment of mental illness related to childbearing has already succeeded in bringing together researchers, health workers and support groups and so provides a most useful forum for professional collaboration.

Clinical psychologists provide a clinical liaison service to obstetric units, as well as to health centres and have contributed substantially to research advances. The growth of the journal associated with the Society for Reproductive and Infant Psychology is firm evidence of this research interest.

The Association of Health visitors and the Royal College of Midwives are also aware of the need to equip their students with the clinical skills to identify postnatal depression, and increasingly recognise that their professions must make a distinctive contribution to the diagnosis and management of this disorder.

Community psychiatric nurses make available their expertise, more especially and perhaps distinctively, in the management and postnatal follow-up of women recovering from a major puerperal psychosis and receiving long-term medication.

It is hoped that these various professional groups will encourage each other to persist with research into puerperal mood disorder, and maintain multiprofessional collaboration; some blurring of professional boundaries being necessary if the questions asked by Marcé and Esquirol a century ago are to be answered. This collaboration will only occur if the professional boundaries between health workers are allowed to overlap, and if continuity of medical care from the antenatal to the postnatal clinic is a high priority.

At the present time the clinical descriptions of puerperal mental illnesses are almost complete, and the considerable frequency of these disorders is more widely recognised. What is lacking, however, is a more definitive understanding of their causes and an evaluation of treatment and of prevention. If these tasks are to be undertaken satisfactorily than, researchers and clinicians must collaborate and listen carefully to the mother's own account of her illness, as well as to her criticisms of postnatal care.

Appendix 1

Development of the Edinburgh Postnatal Depression Scale (PDS)

VALIDATION

The validation study of the 13-item PDS took place at Dedridge Health Centre in Livingston which is a new town 15 miles west of Edinburgh.

A sample of 63 mothers who had recently had a baby took part in the study. Each received a letter inviting her to attend the Health Centre to complete a questionnaire about postnatal depression and to be interviewed by one of the research team. Non-attenders received a second letter, and those who did not reply were telephoned or visited at home.

27 mothers came in reply to our first letter, and a further eight after a second appointment had been given. Nine mothers were visited at home before a suitable appointment could be made; only three refused to participate in the study at all.

A further 14 women were specially referred to us by their own Health Visitor because they had 'problems' and two were attending a psychiatric outpatient department. A third had recently been a psychiatric inpatient and two were referred from a postnatal depression support group in Edinburgh.

The Postnatal Depression Scale was then validated against the Semistructured Psychiatric Interview (SPI) of Goldberg et al (1972).

All the SP1 ratings were discussed with J.C., and any difficult ratings agreed, and the psychiatric diagnosis was arrived at using Research Diagnostic Criteria.

Three mothers did not have a complete SPI, two had already had a full interview by a psychiatrist and the third was too distressed. There was nevertheless sufficient clinical information available from other sources for a psychiatric diagnosis to be made.

Sample characteristics

The mean age of the subjects was 27 years (SD 5.2) and of the babies 4 months (SD 1.5 months); 30% were primigravidae; 40% came from social class III, 33% from, social classes IV and V, 9% from social class II and 3% from social class I. 47 mothers had a normal delivery, eight had forceps, and eight had a caesarean section.

The results of the validation study are shown in Figure 7, which indicates clearly that the PDS distinguished satisfactorily between depressed and non-depressed women. Of the 25 mothers who scored above a cut-off of 16, only four were false positives (three of these four having mild psychiatric morbidity but not depression) and there was only one false negative. The sensitivity was 96% and specificity 91%. Interestingly, the one mother with the 'false negative' score had a definite major depressive illness when she attended as a psychiatric outpatient. She later explained that her husband was present when the PDS was completed and that she did not want him to know how bad she was feeling.

The internal consistency of the PDS items is shown in the correlation matrix (Table 2) and was satisfactory. All correlations between items were statistically significant, and the majority of such correlations ranged between 0.6 and 0.8. The item 'I have enjoyed being a mother' had, surprisingly, the lowest correlation with the other items; the items relating to self-blame and self-harm were also weaker predictors than we had expected them to be.

A factor analysis was carried out to determine whether the scale was homogeneous. Two separate factors then emerged. The first, a 'depression factor', explained 46% of the variance, and the second, which explained much less of the variance (23%), had its highest loadings on the 'mother' item and also included the two irritability items. This finding suggested that the 13-item scale

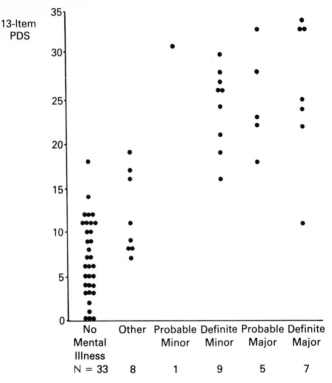

Fig. 7 Validation of 13-item PDS.

could be abbreviated to a 10-item scale without impairing its effectiveness as a screening instrument.

Limitations of the PDS

These results therefore suggest that the PDS is successful in identifying postnatal depression in women at home but does not clearly distinguish between women with a severe and a moderate depression. A further limitation is that the scale only identifies depression and does not detect women with phobias, anxiety neuroses or with obsessive compulsive neuroses. The setting in which the scale is completed is also of the utmost importance if it is to reflect accurately the mother's current mood; a mother is more likely to reveal her true feelings if she completes the scale without being observed closely by others.

Table 2 Correlation matrix of PDS items

	1 Laugh	2 Slam	3 Look forw.	4 Self-blame	5 Anxiety	6 Mother	7 Panic	8 Cope	9 Sleep	10 Sad	11 Hit	12 Cry	13 Self inj.
1 Laugh	1.0	.60	.61	.59	.62	.42	.62	.71	.70	.79	.54	.73	.60
2 Slamming		1.0	.60	.55	.53	.46	.49	.61	.51	.66	.63	.61	.36
3 Look forward			1.0	.49	.52	.37	.62	.68	.69	.63	.55	.66	.58
4 Self-blame				1.0	.62	.26	.53	.57	.50	.59	.47	.48	.33
5 Anxiety					1.0	.28	.79	.67	.53	.69	.46	.68	.48
6 Mother						1.0	.36	.48	.44	.47	.56	.41	.24
7 Panic							1.0	.70	.62	.79	.44	.71	.54
8 Cope								1.0	.74	.76	.61	.77	.55
9 Sleep									1.0	.74	.59	.66	.66
10 Sad										1.0	.65	.82	.65
11 Hit											1.0	.62	.49
12 Cry												1.0	.65
13 Self injury													1.0

The Postnatal Depression Scale does however have satisfactory validity when tested against a psychiatric interview of a community sample of women, and meets other criteria for its usefulness as a screening instrument. Its face validity is most satisfactory and it is fully acceptable to the mothers themselves, as well as to the primary care workers. The PDS may therefore be a useful screening instrument to detect postnatal depression in mothers at a postnatal or a baby clinic.

Our present research shows that the 13-item, or 10-item, PDS is of use in a primary care setting and could make a substantial contribution to the secondary prevention of postnatal depression by facilitating its early detection. It is also likely to be useful in research, but its sensitivity to change over time has not as yet been fully established. We are at present planning to complete our development of the PDS and validate it for use during pregnancy.

Appendix 2

Edinburgh Postnatal Depression Scale: instructions to primary care workers

Postnatal depression is a distressing disorder, more prolonged than the blues which occur in the first week after delivery, but usually less severe than the puerperal psychoses. Previous studies from Edinburgh and elsewhere have shown that postnatal depression occurs in at least 10% of women and that many remain untreated at home. Although a mother with postnatal depression may manage to cope with household tasks, she is nevertheless disadvantaged in other ways and her family can also be adversely affected.

The Edinburgh Postnatal Depression Scale (PDS) has been developed to assist primary care teams to detect such mothers with postnatal depression. The PDS consists of 13 statements which relate to symptoms of postnatal depression. The mother is asked to underline the reply which comes closest to how she has been feeling during the past week. The PDS was developed at baby clinics, and tested at the health centres in Livingston. The validation study showed that mothers who scored 16 or more on the PDS were likely to be suffering from a depressive illness of varying severity and that non-depressed mothers did not usually score above this cut-off point.

INSTRUCTIONS FOR USING THE 13-ITEM PDS

1. The PDS is concerned with how the mother has been feeling during the previous week.

85

2. All 13 items must be completed.
3. The PDS is best administered during the second or third month postpartum; the baby's 6 weeks check-up may well provide a suitable opportunity for its completion.
4. The PDS is a self-report scale, so only in exceptional circumstances, as when a mother has poor understanding of English or difficulty in reading, need the general practitioner or health visitor help with its completion.
5. The PDS should be administered in such a way as to avoid the possibility of the mother discussing her answers with others, as this has been found to influence results. It may be filled in at the clinic, in the surgery or on a home visit, but it should always be handed back immediately on its completion to the doctor or health visitor.
6. Scores for individual items range from 0–3 according to severity. The total score is calculated by adding the scores for each of the 13 PDS items.
7. A score of 16 or more indicates that the mother may be depressed and therefore requires further assessment.

Appendix 3

Postnatal depression: a comparison of African and Scottish women*

INTRODUCTION

Since the risk of puerperal depression is believed to have been enhanced by recent changes in women's roles in Western society and by the increasing likelihood of delivery in hospital, it is sometimes thought that an African woman is relatively unlikely to become depressed in the puerperium. However the small African literature on puerperal psychoses indicates that depressive illness can certainly occur at this time. Ebie (1972) described a series of 60 women with a puerperal psychosis and found 10 to have an affective disorder. Similarly Swift (1972) found 2 out of 40 women with a puerperal psychosis to be depressed, although half of this sample were schizophrenic.

The purpose of this paper is to describe the frequency and symptomatology of puerperal depression in Africans and, by comparison with a similar prospective study of Scottish women, to determine the extent to which socio-cultural factors may modify the symptoms of this disorder.

The study took place at Kasangati Health Centre near Kampala, which was adequately staffed and able to provide comprehensive community services. The mothers mainly belonged to the Ganda

*Cox J L 1983 Social Psychiatry 18:25–28 Reprinted by kind permission of Springer – Verlag, Heidelberg.

tribe. Most families could grow sufficient food because the ground was fertile and rainfall was usually plentiful. The main tasks of Ganda women were to cook, to grow food and to look after their own children and those of others. One-third were co-wives and the extended family usually lived in the same village. One-third of the women were less than 20 years old and their mean age was 24 years.

The 25 villages which formed a defined research area consisted of scattered houses, usually surrounded by banana plantations. Dust tracks connected these villages and were usually passable by car, unless there had been heavy rain. As there were no postal or telephone services, tracing some of the subjects was difficult. However, a mother was only 'lost to follow-up' if three attempts to contact her had failed and neighbours or the village chief had been unable to tell us whether the mother had moved or if she had recently delivered.

The interviews started in June 1972 and were completed in May 1974. At that time Uganda was still peaceful and village life had not yet been disrupted by political changes.

METHOD

Of the 263 women interviewed at the booking-in antenatal visit at the centre, 183 delivered a live baby and formed the sample described in this paper. These 183 women were re-interviewed, usually at home, about 3 months after childbirth. The Luganda modification of the Standardised Psychiatric Interview (SP1:) (Goldberg et al, 1970) was administered by J. C. and a trained Luganda-speaking research assistant. Orley & Wing (1979) report the SPI to have a high correlation with the Present State Examination (Wing et al, 1974) and it was found in general to be satisfactory for the limited descriptive purposes of this study.

The SPI items used in the postnatal interview were similar to those of the antenatal interview, although in the puerperium each symptom was rated for two time periods: the previous 7 days and the time since delivery. The interviewers were always blind to the antenatal psychiatric ratings.

The inter-rater reliability between the author and the research assistant, who spoke both English and Luganda, was satisfactory. Correlations of r = 0.8 were obtained for anxiety and depression scores, while the overall severity score (the sum of the symptom ratings and twice the mental state rating) had a higher correlation of r = 0.9. Any difficult ratings were discussed with the research assistant, and a psychiatric diagnosis agreed using the eighth revision of the International Classification of Disease (ICD 1968). A single diagnosis of depressive illness was made, which included the ICD categories of depressive neurosis and depressive psychosis. In general, the patients with a depressive illness would also have fulfilled Pitt's (1968) criteria for postnatal depression, which included distress to the mother and a duration of at least 2 weeks. Social impairment was rated on a 4-point scale ranging from nil to severe, the latter rating being made if heavy digging or water-carrying had not been possible for at least 6 of the preceding 7 days.

In the prospective Scottish study, which also used the SPI, a representative sample of 89 women were interviewed on four occasions: at their booking-in antenatal clinic, during the third trimester, a week after delivery and 4 months later. A depressive illness was found in 13% of the total sample in the puerperium, compared with 4% during pregnancy; a further 16% subjects reported persistent depressive symptoms following delivery. Full details of this study are presented elsewhere (Cox et al, 1982).

RESULTS

Comparison between the sociocultural characteristics of the 80 African women lost to follow-up and the remaining antenatal sample of 183 showed the former to be more likely to be living alone (P < 0.05), to have been married more recently (P < 0.05) and to have attended the antenatal clinic at more than 35 weeks gestation (P < 0.01). These women were also more likely to have experienced psychiatric symptoms during pregnancy and may therefore have been slightly more at risk of a puerperal psychiatric disorder than those mothers who were successfully re-interviewed.

Psychiatric diagnoses

18 African women (10%) were found to have a depressive illness in the puerperium, usually commencing within 2 weeks of delivery. Of these 18 mothers, six were severely impaired by this

disorder. No association was found between postnatal depression and having a first child or being unmarried. Furthermore, mothers who had delivered their baby in a hospital were not more likely to be depressed than those who had home deliveries. In the interviewed group the mean overall severity score during pregnancy was 10.1 (SD = 11). In the puerperium it was 6.0 (SD = 9.4), a reduction in mean score that was significant at the 0.1% level. The total anxiety, depression and irritability symptoms score was reduced in the puerperium; observed depression and anxiety also showed a significant reduction.

Of the 18 depressed women only four had been depressed during pregnancy, while only four of 18 women with an antenatal depressive illness subsequently developed postnatal depression. In the majority, therefore, postnatal depression was not a continuation of a depressive illness which had begun before delivery. Guilt and self-blame were very rare and described by only two of the total sample interviewed. One mother said others were talking about her and also wondered what she had done to deserve this. The other mother believed that she was bad because she had an epileptic child.

Schizophrenia or organic psychoses were not described in any of the subjects; two had animal phobias — one fearing chameleons and the other caterpillars. Six subjects had an anxiety neurosis.

Comparison with Scottish women

The mean SPI scores for the Africans were then compared with the results of the Scottish study. In general the Africans were observed to be more anxious and depressed than the Scots in pregnancy and more likely to report psychogenic somatic symptoms (fig.8). The frequency of postnatal depression was 10% in the African and 13% in the Scottish sample. There were no differences in most SPI ratings between the Africans and Scots in the puerperium, although only two of the total African sample reported guilt and self-blame in the puerperium compared with at least nine of the Scots.

DISCUSSION

These results need to be interpreted with caution because of the methodological limitations when women from a different culture

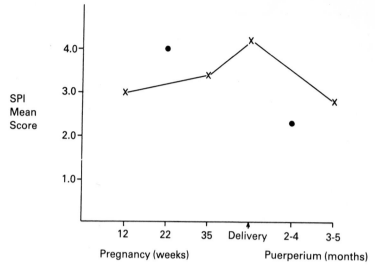

Fig. 8 SP1 mean score (anxiety, depression, irritability) for African women (●): N = 178 and Scottish women (×): N = 89.

to that of the researcher are being interviewed. However, it is clear that postnatal depression is a common disorder in these rural African women and that a traditional way of life and having a home delivery does not reduce the likelihood of this illness. The depressed women were markedly distressed by their symptoms and were also socially impaired; some could not even carry out essential household tasks.

In the majority of women, depression began in the first weeks after childbirth and was not a continuation of a depressive illness that had begun in pregnancy. The frequency of postnatal depression in this study, moreover, is probably an underestimate because women who could not be traced were probably more at risk of a postpartum psychiatric disorder and the medical services in Kasangati were far superior to those available elsewhere.

Although the comparison with the Scottish sample can only be made cautiously, because of the considerable sociocultural differences between the samples, the results do suggest that pregnancy, especially for an African mother, is associated with an anxiety that generally exceeded that observed in the Scottish women. The Africans were more worried at this time about the physical risks of childbirth and often remembered their previous difficult deliveries. Some were even reminded of earlier stillbirths. Thus, although childbearing for an African conferred high status, it was also a time for much apprehension and was certainly not characterised by months of rural contentment. Successful delivery was therefore often associated with a reduction in anxiety; although for some women there was an increased likelihood of becoming depressed at this time. These depressive illnesses, which usually started soon after delivery, were often severe and 10 mothers had marked diurnal variation of mood and early morning wakening.

That the Africans were in general less likely to report guilt or self-blame than the Scots is of interest. The Scots were more likely to be concerned with failure to live up to their expectations of being a 'good mother' derived from their own mother's values or from their observations of friends or neighbours. The Scots were also more likely to question whether or not they were behaving correctly and were particularly concerned if they did not show sufficient affection towards their baby. The Africans by contrast only rarely described such feelings.

Despite these differences of symptoms, the frequency of postnatal depression was surprisingly similar in the two studies. This finding might even suggest that sociocultural factors were less important than biological variables in the aetiology of this disorder, especially as factors such as having a first child or being unmarried, which might increase stress, were not related to an increased likelihood of becoming depressed in either the African or the Scottish samples. Likewise, having a hospital delivery, which could be particularly worrying for an African mother because traditional birth rituals may not be observed, was not found to increase the likelihood of postnatal depression.

The depressed Africans were unlikely to consult a doctor for their symptoms and their relatives may not have regarded them as ill at all. In this respect they were somewhat similar to the Scottish women, who also only rarely consulted a doctor. Traditional healers were probably far more likely to be consulted than doctors by the Ugandans, especially if the mother was thought to have a traditional puerperal mental illness (Cox, 1979).

Little is known about the possible adverse repercussions of postnatal depression on the family and the nutrition of the baby. However, the greater availability of caretaker mothers in Ugandan society may not always compensate for the failure of a severely depressed mother to feed her infant. The findings of this study therefore suggest that maternal and child-health personnel require adequate training in both the recognition and treatment of this common postpartum psychiatric disorder.

REFERENCES

Cox J L 1979 Amakiro: a Ugandan puerperal psychosis? Social Psychiatry 14: 49–52

Cox J L, Connor Y, Kendell R E 1982 Prospective study of the psychiatric disorders of childbirth. British Journal of Psychiatry 140: 111–117

Ebie J C 1972 Psychiatric illness in the puerperium among Nigerians. Tropical Geographical Medicine 24: 253–256

Goldberg D P, Cooper B, Eastwood M R, Kedward H B, Shepherd M 1970 A standardised psychiatric interview for use in community studies. British Journal of Preventive and Social Medicine 24: 18–23

International classification of disease 1968 Her Majesty's Stationery Office, London

Orley J, Wing J K 1979 Psychiatric disorders in two African villages. Archives of General Psychiatry 36: 513–520

Pitt B 1968 'Atypical' depression following childbirth. British Journal of Psychiatry 114: 1325–1335

Swift C R 1972 Psychosis during the puerperium among Tanzanians. East African Medical Journal 49: 651–657

Wing J K, Cooper J E, Sartorius N 1974 The measurement and classification of psychiatric symptoms. Cambridge University Press, Cambridge

Index